Updates on Caries Management in the Primary and Permanent Dentition

Updates on Caries Management in the Primary and Permanent Dentition

Guest Editor
Julian Schmoeckel

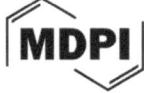

Basel • Beijing • Wuhan • Barcelona • Belgrade • Novi Sad • Cluj • Manchester

Guest Editor
Julian Schmoeckel
Pediatric Dentistry
University Medicine of Greifswald
Greifswald
Germany

Editorial Office
MDPI AG
Grosspeteranlage 5
4052 Basel, Switzerland

This is a reprint of the Special Issue, published open access by the journal *Medicina* (ISSN 1648-9144), freely accessible at: https://www.mdpi.com/journal/medicina/special_issues/7LO70687LS.

For citation purposes, cite each article independently as indicated on the article page online and as indicated below:

Lastname, A.A.; Lastname, B.B. Article Title. *Journal Name* **Year**, *Volume Number*, Page Range.

ISBN 978-3-7258-3407-5 (Hbk)
ISBN 978-3-7258-3408-2 (PDF)
https://doi.org/10.3390/books978-3-7258-3408-2

© 2025 by the authors. Articles in this book are Open Access and distributed under the Creative Commons Attribution (CC BY) license. The book as a whole is distributed by MDPI under the terms and conditions of the Creative Commons Attribution-NonCommercial-NoDerivs (CC BY-NC-ND) license (https://creativecommons.org/licenses/by-nc-nd/4.0/).

Contents

Julian Schmoeckel
Updates on Caries Management in the Primary and Permanent Dentition
Reprinted from: *Medicina* 2025, *61*, 316, https://doi.org/10.3390/medicina61020316 1

Bakr A. Rashid, Ahmad Al Masri, Christian H. Splieth, Mustafa Abdalla and Julian Schmoeckel
Dental Decision-Making in Pediatric Dentistry: A Cross-Sectional Case-Based Questionnaire Among Dentists in Germany
Reprinted from: *Medicina* 2024, *60*, 1907, https://doi.org/10.3390/medicina60111907 4

Sandra Petrauskienė, Kristina Saldūnaitė-Mikučionienė and Julija Narbutaitė
Survival Analysis of Glass Ionomer Cement and Resin-Based Sealant Retention: A 10-Year Follow-Up Study
Reprinted from: *Medicina* 2024, *60*, 756, https://doi.org/10.3390/medicina60050756 19

Diego González-Gil, Javier Flores-Fraile, Vicente Vera-Rodríguez, Andrea Martín-Vacas and Joaquín López-Marcos
Comparative Meta-Analysis of Minimally Invasive and Conventional Approaches for Caries Removal in Permanent Dentition
Reprinted from: *Medicina* 2024, *60*, 402, https://doi.org/10.3390/medicina60030402 31

Yoko Asahi, Katsuaki Naito, Hikaru Kanda, Kazuaki Niwano, Daisuke Takegawa, Hiromichi Yumoto, et al.
Clinical Investigation of the Inhibitory Effects of Tooth-Coating Materials on Initial Active Root Caries: A Pilot Randomized Controlled Trial
Reprinted from: *Medicina* 2024, *60*, 150, https://doi.org/10.3390/medicina60010150 42

Ruba Abdulrahim, Christian H. Splieth, Mhd Said Mourad, Annina Vielhauer, Manasi R. Khole and Ruth M. Santamaría
Silver Diamine Fluoride Renaissance in Paediatric Dentistry: A 24-Month Retrospective and Cross-Sectional Analysis
Reprinted from: *Medicina* 2024, *60*, 16, https://doi.org/10.3390/medicina60010016 54

Mohamed Abudrya, Christian H. Splieth, Mhd Said Mourad and Ruth M. Santamaría
Efficacy of Different Fluoride Therapies on Hypersensitive Carious Lesions in Primary Teeth
Reprinted from: *Medicina* 2023, *59*, 2042, https://doi.org/10.3390/medicina59112042 65

Demetrio Lamloum, Marco Dettori, Pino La Corte, Maria Ruth Agnoli, Andrea Cappai, Arianna Viarchi, et al.
Oral Health Survey in Burundi; Evaluation of the Caries Experience in Schoolchildren Using the DMFT Index
Reprinted from: *Medicina* 2023, *59*, 1538, https://doi.org/10.3390/medicina59091538 78

Claudia Tighiceanu, Elena Raluca Bulai, Oana Camelia Iatcu, Constantin Dulucheanu and Alexandru Nemtoi
Effect of Vegetable Juices on Properties of Two Resin Composites Used for Dental Caries Management
Reprinted from: *Medicina* 2023, *59*, 774, https://doi.org/10.3390/medicina59040774 88

Eilaf E. A. Ahmed, Salma Al Nesser and Julian Schmoeckel
Introducing an Innovative Approach for Managing Proximal Non-Cavitated Carious Lesions in Juvenile Permanent Dentition: Combining Orthodontic Separators and Silver Fluoride Application
Reprinted from: *Medicina* **2023**, *59*, 1892, https://doi.org/10.3390/medicina59111892 . . . . **98**

Thomas Gerhard Wolf and Guglielmo Campus
Cost-Effectiveness of Treatment Decisions for Early Childhood Caries in Infants and Toddlers: A Systematic Review
Reprinted from: *Medicina* **2023**, *59*, 1865, https://doi.org/10.3390/medicina59101865 . . . . **112**

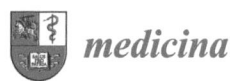

Editorial

Updates on Caries Management in the Primary and Permanent Dentition

Julian Schmoeckel

Department of Pediatric Dentistry, University Medicine Greifswald, 17489 Greifswald, Germany; julian.schmoeckel@uni-greifswald.de

Caries is still one of the most prevalent diseases affecting children and adults worldwide [1]. Reducing its prevalence and improving the quality of dental care, along with the oral-health-related quality of life, should, therefore, be a major goal.

The aim of this Special Issue was to present innovative approaches, high-quality clinical, epidemiological, and dental public health research, or translational research on several aspects of the management of dental caries (preventive/non-invasive, minimally invasive, operative approaches) in children and adults.

First of all, I would like to emphasise that this Special Issue contains a variety of study types, reflecting the different options in research methodology: meta-analysis, systematic reviews, epidemiological research, laboratory studies, retrospective and prospective clinical studies, RCTs, and innovative case series. Furthermore, the Special Issue includes articles on the management of caries in primary teeth and permanent teeth, as well as root caries. This demonstrates the different approaches and perspectives in cariology.

I am delighted that this completed Special Issue contains interesting innovations relating to this topic. In the following, I would like to summarise and highlight specific aspects of the contents of this Special Issue and give my personal outlook for the future.

An epidemiological study on oral health in children in Burundi showed a significant level of caries experience and a very low treatment index, highlighting that caries treatment does not reach the children [2]. This underlines the importance of improvements in prevention and easily assessable and inexpensive management options.

The number of papers in this Special Issue dealing with silver fluoride (SDF) products shows that this is a hot topic and should not be seen as an unsatisfying compromise for so-called "third-world countries" but as a viable alternative or synergistic option for caries management at any stage and on any tooth surface in any patient worldwide.

To my knowledge, two of the published papers [3,4] are related to award-winning presentations at the ORCA Congress 2023 [3] and 2024 [5]. Interestingly, both deal with the use of silver fluoride: (1) in primary teeth, which may eventually dramatically reduce the need for dental general anaesthesia [6], and (2) for young permanent teeth, providing the first pilot data of a reported innovative approach to managing non-cavitated proximal caries [5]. This provides new insights into the potential of silver diamine fluoride (SDF) for treatment of early childhood caries (ECC) [7], as well as options for the management of proximal caries that go beyond the findings from a recent systematic review and meta-analysis [8]. In addition, a double cohort study comparing SDF and 5% fluoride varnish showed that both materials reduced hypersensitivity in children with ECC, but that the potential for caries arrest was much higher with SDF [9].

A laboratory study has shown that an individual's diet may influence the colour stability and microhardness of composite restorations, which are probably one of the most common treatment approaches for caries worldwide [10].

Received: 18 December 2024
Revised: 20 January 2025
Accepted: 21 January 2025
Published: 11 February 2025

Citation: Schmoeckel, J. Updates on Caries Management in the Primary and Permanent Dentition. *Medicina* **2025**, *61*, 316. https://doi.org/10.3390/medicina61020316

Copyright: © 2025 by the author. Published by MDPI on behalf of the Lithuanian University of Health Sciences. Licensee MDPI, Basel, Switzerland. This article is an open access article distributed under the terms and conditions of the Creative Commons Attribution (CC BY) license (https://creativecommons.org/licenses/by/4.0/).

A long-term split-mouth clinical study from Lithuania compared the survival rate of resin-based and GIC-based fissure sealants and showed that their effectiveness in preventing fissure caries in permanent second molars did not differ significantly over a 10-year follow-up period [11].

A meta-analysis of RCTs on the selective caries removal technique in permanent teeth also confirms, in line with another earlier consensus from ORCA [12,13], that selective caries removal is a less invasive approach to pulp tissue perseveration compared with conventional "complete caries removal" techniques [14].

A fairly wide-ranging systematic review on the cost-effectiveness of ECC treatment shows that socio-economic, cultural, and ethnic differences need to be taken into account [15]. This is particularly important in populations with a high prevalence of ECC and with a highly polarised distribution of ECC, in order to implement the most cost-effective approaches.

The direction of minimally invasive dentistry is also favoured by the authors of a study on root caries [16], which shows that the progression of initial active root carious lesions using GICs may be an interesting and promising approach.

Last but not least, a study on decision making for caries management in children shows that this part is much more complex than a tooth-level decision. Consequently, there is a need for simple and effective treatments, while unfortunately, there is still a tendency for too invasive or unrecommended treatment suggestions. The main challenge is to always make the correct diagnosis based on appropriate examinations (clinical, radiographic, etc.). Perhaps future innovations in artificial intelligence will assist dentists in facilitating diagnosis, and robots will be able to perform the necessary restorations or procedures.

I am confident that in the future, with continued research and development of novel treatment strategies, further reductions in the caries prevalence in all age groups worldwide will be achieved. Personalised medicine, multimodal and interdisciplinary management, and digital innovations can further transform the way in which we approach the field of cariology, both clinically and scientifically. Several aspects in the field of caries management have been addressed in research, but there are still relevant gaps, mainly in the areas of research on cost-effectiveness and the translation of knowledge into everyday dental practice. These advances will bring us closer to our goal of improving the oral-health-related quality of life of millions of children, adolescents, adults, and seniors.

Conflicts of Interest: The author declares no conflicts of interest.

References

1. Kassebaum, N.J.; Bernabé, E.; Dahiya, M.; Bhandari, B.; Murray, C.J.L.; Marcenes, W. Global burden of untreated caries: A systematic review and metaregression. *J. Dent. Res.* **2015**, *94*, 650–658. [CrossRef] [PubMed]
2. Lamloum, D.; Dettori, M.; La Corte, P.; Agnoli, M.R.; Cappai, A.; Viarchi, A.; Arghittu, A.; Wolf, T.G.; Castiglia, P.; Campus, G. Oral Health Survey in Burundi; Evaluation of the Caries Experience in Schoolchildren Using the DMFT Index. *Medicina* **2023**, *59*, 1538. [CrossRef] [PubMed]
3. Abdulrahim, R.; Splieth, C.H.; Mourad, M.S.; Vielhauer, A.; Khole, M.R.; Santamaría, R.M. Silver Diamine Fluoride Renaissance in Paediatric Dentistry: A 24-Month Retrospective and Cross-Sectional Analysis. *Medicina* **2023**, *60*, 16. [CrossRef] [PubMed]
4. Ahmed, E.E.A.; Al Nesser, S.; Schmoeckel, J. Introducing an Innovative Approach for Managing Proximal Non-Cavitated Carious Lesions in Juvenile Permanent Dentition: Combining Orthodontic Separators and Silver Fluoride Application. *Medicina* **2023**, *59*, 1892. [CrossRef] [PubMed]
5. Ahmed, E.E.A.; Al Nesser, S.; Mourad, M.S.; Splieth, C.H.; Schmoeckel, J. Innovative management of multiple non-cavitated proximal caries in high-risk patients: Combining SDF & orthodontic separators. In *71st ORCA Congress*; Karger: Basel, Switzerland, 2024; p. 196. [CrossRef]
6. Abdulrahim, R.; Splieth, C.H.; Mourad, M.S.; Vielhauer, A.; Santamaría, R.M. Impact of Silver Diammine Fluoride Use on the Need for Dental General Anaesthesia Treatment in Children. In *70th ORCA Congress*; Karger: Basel, Switzerland, 2023; p. 381.
7. Schmoeckel, J.; Gorseta, K.; Splieth, C.H.; Juric, H. How to Intervene in the Caries Process: Early Childhood Caries-A Systematic Review. *Caries Res.* **2020**, *54*, 102–112. [CrossRef] [PubMed]

8. Splieth, C.H.; Kanzow, P.; Wiegand, A.; Schmoeckel, J.; Jablonski-Momeni, A. How to intervene in the caries process: Proximal caries in adolescents and adults-a systematic review and meta-analysis. *Clin. Oral Investig.* **2020**, *24*, 1623–1636. [CrossRef] [PubMed]
9. Abudrya, M.; Splieth, C.H.; Mourad, M.S.; Santamaría, R.M. Efficacy of Different Fluoride Therapies on Hypersensitive Carious Lesions in Primary Teeth. *Medicina* **2023**, *59*, 2042. [CrossRef] [PubMed]
10. Tighiceanu, C.; Bulai, E.R.; Iatcu, O.C.; Dulucheanu, C.; Nemtoi, A. Effect of Vegetable Juices on Properties of Two Resin Composites Used for Dental Caries Management. *Medicina* **2023**, *59*, 774. [CrossRef] [PubMed]
11. Petrauskienė, S.; Saldūnaitė-Mikučionienė, K.; Narbutaitė, J. Survival Analysis of Glass Ionomer Cement and Resin-Based Sealant Retention: A 10-Year Follow-Up Study. *Medicina* **2024**, *60*, 756. [CrossRef] [PubMed]
12. Splieth, C.H.; Banerjee, A.; Bottenberg, P.; Breschi, L.; Campus, G.; Ekstrand, K.R.; Giacaman, R.A.; Haak, R.; Hannig, M.; Hickel, R.; et al. How to Intervene in the Caries Process in Children: A Joint ORCA and EFCD Expert Delphi Consensus Statement. *Caries Res.* **2020**, *54*, 297–305. [CrossRef] [PubMed]
13. Machiulskiene, V.; Campus, G.; Carvalho, J.C.; Dige, I.; Ekstrand, K.R.; Jablonski-Momeni, A.; Maltz, M.; Manton, D.J.; Martignon, S.; Martinez-Mier, E.A.; et al. Terminology of Dental Caries and Dental Caries Management: Consensus Report of a Workshop Organized by ORCA and Cariology Research Group of IADR. *Caries Res.* **2020**, *54*, 7–14. [CrossRef] [PubMed]
14. González-Gil, D.; Flores-Fraile, J.; Vera-Rodríguez, V.; Martín-Vacas, A.; López-Marcos, J. Comparative Meta-Analysis of Minimally Invasive and Conventional Approaches for Caries Removal in Permanent Dentition. *Medicina* **2024**, *60*, 402. [CrossRef] [PubMed]
15. Wolf, T.G.; Campus, G. Cost-Effectiveness of Treatment Decisions for Early Childhood Caries in Infants and Toddlers: A Systematic Review. *Medicina* **2023**, *59*, 1865. [CrossRef] [PubMed]
16. Asahi, Y.; Naito, K.; Kanda, H.; Niwano, K.; Takegawa, D.; Yumoto, H.; Noiri, Y.; Hayashi, M. Clinical Investigation of the Inhibitory Effects of Tooth-Coating Materials on Initial Active Root Caries: A Pilot Randomized Controlled Trial. *Medicina* **2024**, *60*, 150. [CrossRef] [PubMed]

Disclaimer/Publisher's Note: The statements, opinions and data contained in all publications are solely those of the individual author(s) and contributor(s) and not of MDPI and/or the editor(s). MDPI and/or the editor(s) disclaim responsibility for any injury to people or property resulting from any ideas, methods, instructions or products referred to in the content.

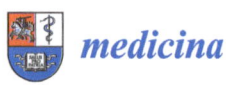

Article

Dental Decision-Making in Pediatric Dentistry: A Cross-Sectional Case-Based Questionnaire Among Dentists in Germany

Bakr A. Rashid [1], Ahmad Al Masri [1,2], Christian H. Splieth [1], Mustafa Abdalla [3] and Julian Schmoeckel [1,*]

1. Department of Pediatric Dentistry, University Medicine Greifswald, Walther-Rathenau Str. 42a, 17475 Greifswald, Germany; bakr.rashid@stud.uni-greifswald.de (B.A.R.); ahmad.almasri@uni-greifswald.de (A.A.M.); splieth@uni-greifswald.de (C.H.S.)
2. Department of Orthodontics, University Medicine Greifswald, Walther-Rathenau Str. 42a, 17475 Greifswald, Germany
3. MyPediaClinic, Dubai Healthcare City, Dubai P.O. Box 505206, United Arab Emirates; drmustafaabdalla@hotmail.com
* Correspondence: julian.schmoeckel@uni-greifswald.de; Tel.: +49-383-486-7167

Citation: Rashid, B.A.; Al Masri, A.; Splieth, C.H.; Abdalla, M.; Schmoeckel, J. Dental Decision-Making in Pediatric Dentistry: A Cross-Sectional Case-Based Questionnaire Among Dentists in Germany. *Medicina* **2024**, *60*, 1907. https://doi.org/10.3390/medicina60111907

Academic Editor: Gaetano Isola

Received: 18 October 2024
Revised: 13 November 2024
Accepted: 18 November 2024
Published: 20 November 2024

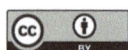

Copyright: © 2024 by the authors. Published by MDPI on behalf of the Lithuanian University of Health Sciences. Licensee MDPI, Basel, Switzerland. This article is an open access article distributed under the terms and conditions of the Creative Commons Attribution (CC BY) license (https://creativecommons.org/licenses/by/4.0/).

Abstract: *Background and Objectives*: The most recent guidelines and recommendations regarding treatments of dental caries in children are shifting towards evidence-based minimal or non-invasive approaches aiming to preserve the vitality of teeth and potentially reduce the need for dental general anesthesia. This study investigated the treatment recommendations of dentists actively practicing pediatric dentistry in Germany regarding different patient cases with caries in primary teeth. *Materials and Methods*: The questionnaire was distributed on paper or online to pediatric dentists and general dentists practicing pediatric dentistry. Five cases of children with dental treatment needs representing a variety of clinical situations were selected for the questionnaire. Considering four different scenarios regarding pain symptoms (yes/no) and cooperation level (good/low) for each case resulted in 20 questions, where the preferred treatment option could be chosen out of 21 options ranging from observation only to extraction with/without different sedation techniques. The answers were categorized into three categories for each case and scenario according to guidelines, recent scientific evidence, and recommendations (recommended, acceptable, or not recommended/contraindicated). *Results*: In total, 222 participants responded to the survey (161 female; 72.5%). In 55.2% of the total 4440 answers, the participants chose a "recommended" treatment option, in 16.4% "acceptable", but in 28.4%, a "not recommended" treatment, which ranged for the five cases between 18.7 and 36.1%. While pain and low cooperation levels led to more invasive and justified treatment choices (only 26.3% "not recommended"), less severe scenarios resulted more often in "not recommended" options (pain with good cooperation: 31.0%; or low cooperation without pain: 32.6%). The dentist's age, experience, and educational background did not significantly correlate to choosing "not recommended" treatment options. *Conclusions*: A child's pain and cooperation level greatly impact the treatment decisions made by dentists, with a risk of too-invasive treatment options in low-severity cases. Substantial disparities in treatment recommendations for caries in primary teeth persist among dental practitioners regardless of their age, experience, and educational background.

Keywords: dentistry; primary teeth; dental treatment; decision-making; nitrous oxide sedation; general anesthesia

1. Introduction

Decision-making in medicine and dentistry is one of the most critical steps before initiating any clinical treatment. Especially in pediatric dentistry, many factors should be considered in the process of decision-making, far beyond tooth level, such as the cooperation level of the child, the overall oral treatment need, caries risk and activity, the accuracy of the diagnosis, potential risks of the treatment and sedation options, the financial aspects, and the duration of the treatment [1–3]. In modern dentistry, reaching a treatment decision is not done by the dentist alone (anymore). A change from the traditional, rather so-called "paternalistic" approach to more participative approaches with informed consent has occurred in medicine and dentistry in the past decades [4], which is oriented toward the autonomy of the patients and includes their competencies. Pediatric health care has the challenge of having "immature" patients with limited cooperation and understanding of health issues, as well as difficulties regarding parental preferences. This makes decision-making in pediatric dentistry far more challenging than other specialties in dentistry, which should not be underestimated, as the initial recommendations of the dentist for a certain treatment path lay the basis for later communication and decision-making with informed consent from the parent or the guardian [3].

The challenges in decision-making in pediatric dentistry extend beyond finding the balance between parental preferences and children's capabilities, as the treatment options on the tooth level have witnessed a shift towards minimal or non-invasive approaches. The conventional restoration (CR) of a cavity on a primary tooth using amalgam, glass ionomer cement, resin composite, or polyacrylic acid-modified composites used to be the standard treatment in pediatric dentistry [5]. These types of restorations are still widely used, even though they show weak performance with a high need for retreatment [6] and may be associated with a high risk of restoration failure and pulpal complications [7]. With a correct pulp diagnosis of reversible pulpitis, selective carious tissue removal or caries sealing (e.g., the Hall technique) could be performed, avoiding complete caries removal near the pulp and minimizing the risk of pulp exposure, which can preserve the vitality of the primary molar [8]. Non-restorative cavity control (NRCC) is also a modern concept that aims to arrest the progression of caries through oral hygiene after removing overhanging enamel and dentin, if needed, to make the lesion accessible, which should be followed by repeated and regular biofilm removal as well as fluoride application to stimulate the remineralization of the carious tooth structure and stop the activity of the lesion arresting its progression, which requires the high adherence of patients and/or parents to manage the lesion [2]. The integration of silver diamine fluoride (SDF) and the Hall technique (HT) into modern caries management in pediatric dentistry has expanded the dental treatment spectrum in pediatric dentistry and provided options for children with limited cooperation, offering effective solutions with minimal invasiveness. These evidence-based approaches provide comprehensive care while prioritizing the preservation of tooth structure and patient comfort [9–11]. Moreover, sedation methods such as nitrous oxide or general anesthesia (GA) widen the spectrum of treatment approaches even further, which makes the decision on the best treatment approach in different circumstances in pediatric dentistry even more challenging. In general, no single treatment option is the only possible, and no treatment option can always be considered the best. However, some good treatment options might be considered unsatisfactory in certain circumstances or situations. For instance, a pulpotomy on a symptomless primary tooth with (deep) proximal dentin caries is an evidence-based approach with reported high success rates. Still, in a case of low cooperation, the treatment would probably require sedation or even GA. Considering the risks of GA along with other less invasive evidence-based approaches, such as the HT with a diagnosis of reversible pulpitis, a pulpotomy could be considered disadvantageous as the HT is possible even in the case of limited cooperation, avoiding the need for DGA [12].

With these wide ranges of treatment options and approaches in pediatric dentistry and the shift towards minimal and non-invasive treatments, it remains unclear whether daily clinical practices are following the updates in the literature. Therefore, this study aimed to investigate the treatment recommendations of dentists actively practicing pediatric dentistry in Germany based on different cases of caries in primary dentition, with suggested scenarios considering pain symptoms and cooperation levels.

2. Materials and Methods

This questionnaire-based study includes five cases with clinical and/or radiographical pictures suggesting different dental treatment options with different scenarios.

2.1. Study Population and Data Collection

As the study aimed to investigate the different approaches of dentists in different clinical scenarios and cases in pediatric dentistry, it was necessary to include a large number of participants actively practicing pediatric dentistry, regardless of their qualifications and specialization. The questionnaire was sent via email to all listed pediatric dental clinics from the website of the German Society for Pediatric Dentistry (DGKiZ, N = 360) and to all participants in, as well as graduates of, a postgraduate master's program in Preventive and Pediatric Dentistry at the University of Greifswald in Germany (N = 108). Moreover, the questionnaire was handed out personally to general dentists in Germany (N = 86) who were attending continuing education courses in the field of pediatric dentistry before the start of the course to avoid bias. To calculate the sample size, the population size of dentists practicing pediatric dentistry was anticipated to be around 3500. With a 95% confidence interval and a 10% margin of error, a sample size of 94 was needed. Data collection was done in the period from March 2020 to August 2022.

2.2. The Questionnaire

A questionnaire was designed to include five typical cases of dental caries in primary teeth with clinical and/or radiographical pictures. Participants were asked to choose their recommended treatment option for each case 4 times for different scenarios that reflect real-life scenarios in pediatric dentistry. The four scenarios for each case were as follows:

- No reported pain, cooperative child   (P−, ↑);
- No reported pain, uncooperative child   (P−, ↓);
- Reported pain symptoms, cooperative child   (P+, ↑);
- Reported pain symptoms, uncooperative child (P+, ↓).

The predefined treatment options for the cases with the different scenarios in the survey were 20 in total. They ranged from observation to invasive treatment options such as endodontic treatment or extraction of the tooth, considering also the treatment setting, such as nitrous oxide sedation or GA. The participants had an extra space after each question for typing a treatment option other than the listed ones. Traditional treatment options such as complete caries removal and filling and modern, less traditional treatment modalities such as silver diamine fluoride (SDF) and the Hall technique (HT) were all included as options. An overview of the treatment options and the cases can be seen in Table 1.

The five selected cases included a range of clinical situations concerning children with dental treatment needs, which covered most of the problems and challenges in caries management in primary teeth (Table 1):

- **Case 1:** arrested deep carious lesions (ICDAS 6) on first primary molars (74, 84) in a preschool child;
- **Case 2:** active deep proximal carious lesion (ICDAS 5) on a second primary molar (85) in a preschool child with high caries experience;
- **Case 3:** proximal carious lesion on a first primary molar (74, likely ICDAS 4, detected in bitewing radiograph as D2 lesion) in an elementary schoolchild;
- **Case 4:** clinical and periapical X-ray showing a proximal ICDAS 5 lesion and an occlusal ICDAS 4 lesion on a second primary molar with a dentine bridge between the lesion and the pulp in a preschool child;
- **Case 5:** clinical picture of semi-active dentine carious lesions on anterior primary teeth (Early Childhood Caries; 3-year-old child).

Table 1. The cases and scenarios along with the percentage-wise assignment of each treatment option to the categories of level of recommendation (colors), and the results of the participants in percentages (n = 222).

Cases	Case 1 Arrested ICDAS 6 on #74 and #84				Case 2 Active ICDAS 5 #85				Case 3 ICDAS 4 Proximal #74				Case 4 ICDAS 4 Okklusal and ICDAS 5 Proximal #65				Case 5 ECC #52–62			
	P−↑	P−↓	P+↑	P+↓	P−↑	P−↓	P+↑	P+↓	P−↑	P−↓	P+↑	P+↓	P−↑	P−↓	P+↑	P+↓	P−↑	P−↓	P+↑	P+↓
Treatment options/different scenarios *																				
No treatment/observation only	2.7	6.3	-	1.4	-	3.2	-	1.8	0.9	4.5	0.5	2.7	0.9	1.8	0.5	2.7	0.9	4.5	2.7	3.6
Non-restorative caries control: fluoride varnish and brushing instructions	10.8	30.6	-	0.5	1.8	8.6	-	2.7	2.7	18.0	0.9	6.3	2.7	10.4	0.5	1.8	15.3	24.8	1.4	3.2
Silver diamine fluoride application	2.3	19.4	0.5	5.0	1.4	24.8	0.5	4.1	1.4	14.0	0.9	8.6	0.9	20.7	1.4	4.1	17.1	34.2	6.3	7.2
Atraumatic restorative treatment with glass ionomer filling (ART)	3.6	4.5	2.7	3.6	1.8	9.0	2.3	6.8	1.8	3.6	2.3	2.7	2.3	9.5	2.3	2.7	3.2	4.1	1.8	0.9
GIC filling (with complete caries removal)	2.7	1.4	1.8	1.4	5.9	2.7	4.1	2.3	4.5	3.2	3.2	1.8	3.6	3.2	1.8	2.3	0.5	0.5	-	0.9
Compomer filling (selective caries removal)	15.3	2.7	6.8	1.4	19.4	2.3	4.5	1.4	23.0	5.9	14.0	2.7	15.8	3.6	6.8	0.5	11.7	1.8	7.2	0.5
Compomer filling (complete caries removal)	8.1	-	4.5	-	17.1	0.9	8.6	0.5	33.8	8.1	19.8	5.4	25.2	3.6	6.3	0.5	3.3	0.5	2.3	-
Zirconia pediatric crown	0.5	-	0.9	-	-	-	-	-	-	-	-	-	-	-	-	0.5	9.9	5.4	5.9	3.6
Strip crown composite restoration	-	-	-	-	-	-	-	-	0.5	-	0.5	-	-	-	-	-	28.8	6.3	10.4	2.3
Stainless steel crown (SSC) in Hall technique (no caries removal, no preparation)	24.8	13.5	1.4	1.8	13.5	15.3	2.7	3.6	12.2	19.8	6.8	11.7	16.2	14.0	1.4	0.5	0.5	0.5	0.5	0.9
SSC in conventional technique (complete caries removal, preparation)	8.6	0.9	1.8	0.5	10.8	1.8	6.8	0.9	7.7	1.4	5.9	0.9	6.8	1.8	5.9	0.9	-	-	0.5	-
Pulpotomy and SSC	11.7	1.4	37.4	1.4	18.9	0.9	36.9	-	7.7	-	26.1	2.3	19.4	0.9	39.6	2.3	-	-	1.8	-
Pulpotomy and SSC with nitrous oxide sedation	4.5	3.6	6.8	15.8	4.5	7.7	8.6	19.4	1.4	9.5	8.1	16.7	3.2	11.3	9.0	21.2	0.5	-	0.9	-
Pulpotomy and SSC under general anesthesia	0.5	8.1	3.6	19.4	2.7	17.6	2.7	25.2	0.5	8.1	1.8	20.3	0.9	14.9	1.8	23.9	0.5	0.9	1.8	2.7
Calcium hydroxide/iodoform paste, pulpectomy, and SSC	1.4	-	8.6	-	1.4	0.5	10.4	0.5	0.9	0.5	3.6	-	1.4	0.5	9.5	0.9	-	0.5	4.5	-
Calcium hydroxide/iodoform paste, pulpectomy, and SSC with nitrous oxide sedation	-	0.9	4.1	5.0	-	0.5	2.7	6.3	-	0.5	0.9	4.1	0.5	1.4	4.5	7.7	-	0.5	0.9	4.5
Calcium hydroxide/iodoform paste, pulpectomy, and SSC under general anesthesia	0.5	0.9	0.5	7.7	0.5	2.3	1.8	7.7	1.4	3.2	1.4	4.5	-	1.8	1.4	9.5	0.9	1.4	3.6	7.2
Local anesthesia extraction	1.8	-	12.2	0.5	-	0.5	3.6	0.9	-	-	1.8	-	-	-	5.4	0.9	2.3	0.9	16.7	2.3
Local anesthesia extraction with nitrous oxide sedation	0.5	1.4	5.9	9.5	0.5	0.5	3.2	5.0	-	-	1.4	5.0	-	-	2.3	6.8	-	2.3	14.0	7.7
Extraction under general anesthesia	-	4.5	0.9	25.7	-	1.4	0.9	11.3	-	-	0.5	4.5	0.5	0.9	-	10.8	5.5	11.3	17.1	52.7
Percentage of chosen recommended treatment options	71.6	74.3	74.8	52.7	59.5	57.7	65.3	49.1	76.6	19.8	34.2	11.7	58.1	45.0	70.3	50.9	83.8	63.5	30.6	52.7
Percentage of chosen possible and acceptable treatment options	13.1	3.6	5.0	30.2	1.8	25.2	7.7	36.0	13.1	41.4	48.2	33.8	-	-	-	31.1	3.2	6.3	8.1	19.8
Percentage of chosen not recommended or contraindicated treatment options	15.3	22.1	20.3	17.1	38.7	17.1	27.0	14.9	10.4	38.7	17.6	54.5	41.9	55	29.7	18	13.1	30.2	61.3	27.5

Green colored: Recommended treatment. Yellow colored: Acceptable treatment. Red colored: Not recommended/contraindicated treatment. * Abbreviations and symbols: ↑: cooperative child, ↓: uncooperative Child, P+: pain symptoms, P−: no pain symptoms, ART: atraumatic restorative treatment, ECC: Early Childhood Caries, GIC: glass ionomer cement, ICDAS: International Caries Detection and Assessment System, SSC: stainless steel crown.

All the cases and questions focused on a specific tooth, and not on all carious teeth in the pictures because patient-level decisions are much more complicated and require a thorough explanation for many related factors, which would lengthen the questionnaire and the time required to fill it out and thus reduce the response rate. However, patient-related aspects were still considered in the scenarios mentioned above, mainly regarding pain symptoms and the cooperation level of the child. Other relevant information on the patient level is obtainable from the given pictures/radiographs, such as caries experience/risk/activity and phase of dentition.

Moreover, to investigate the factors influencing dental decision-making, the demographic data of the participants were collected, as well as answers to further questions regarding the number of children treated per week, years of experience as a dentist, years of experience with nitrous oxide sedation and GA, and years of practice as a specialist in pediatric dentistry.

2.3. Ethical Considerations

This study was conducted in full conformance with the principles of the "Declaration of Helsinki" and Good Clinical Practice (GCP) and within the laws and regulations of Greifswald University. Whether on the paper form or online, informed consent was obtained from all participants before filling out the questionnaire. Ethical approval was obtained from the Ethical Committee of the University of Greifswald (BB 052/20). The clinical intra-oral pictures of the patients were presented anonymously to study participants, as consent was taken from the parents/guardians of the children to use the intra-oral photos and/or X-rays in anonymous form for research purposes.

2.4. Treatment Recommendations

Three specialists in pediatric dentistry from the University of Greifswald met to develop an outline for rating the treatment options for the different cases with consideration of the scenarios; two of the three were specialist pediatric dentists and members of the university teaching staff with clinical experience, while the third was a last year postgraduate student in a master program in Preventive and Pediatric Dentistry. A fourth specialist pediatric dentist, who was the head of the Department of Preventive and Pediatric Dentistry at the university and of the mentioned master's program, with a leading role in many worldwide recognized organizations in the field of cariology and pediatric dentistry, was consulted for his opinion in the treatment recommendations. The decision on categorizing the treatment options was thus based on the actual international recommendations and guidelines, yet with consideration of clinical real-life experience. The treatment options were divided according to the case and the suggested scenario into the following categories:

- **Recommended treatment options:** treatment options that follow the up-to-date evidence-based recommendations and guidelines for the management of the mentioned tooth/teeth, considering the suggested scenario regarding pain symptoms and the cooperation level of the child;
- **Possible and acceptable treatment options:** treatment options that do not follow the up-to-date evidence-based recommendations and guidelines for the management of the mentioned tooth/teeth, considering the suggested scenario regarding pain symptoms and the cooperation level of the child. However, although these treatment options are not up-to-date, they are still not contraindicated and could be performed;
- **Not recommended and contraindicated treatment options:** treatment options that do not follow the up-to-date evidence-based recommendations and guidelines for managing the mentioned tooth/teeth, considering the suggested scenario regarding pain symptoms and the cooperation level of the child, which are disadvantageous or even contraindicated.

2.5. Statistical Analysis

The questionnaire responses were exported to an Excel sheet (Microsoft Office 2021), anonymously coded, assigned to the categories of recommendation level as in Table 1, and exported into IBM SPSS for Windows (Version 23.0) for analysis. Frequencies and percentages were calculated for all qualitative variables, while means and standard deviations (SDs) were computed for quantitative variables. To investigate the factors influencing dental decision-making, the number of chosen "not recommended and contraindicated" treatment options was analyzed as the dependent variable. The independent variables considered were age, years of experience as a dentist, experience with nitrous oxide (in years), experience with general anesthesia (in years), years of practicing as a specialist, and the number of children treated per week.

A negative binomial regression model was used to investigate the factors that might lead to choosing an increased number of contraindicated treatment options. A further analysis was performed for each of the independent variables separately to investigate if any of these variables would show an effect on the total numbers of selected "not recommended/contraindicated" treatment options, where a Mann–Whitney test was performed for the categorial variables and Pearson correlation was used for the continuous variables. Moreover, a chi-square analysis was performed to analyze the differences in the distribution of the answers to the three categories of recommendation level between the cases and the scenarios. Statistical significance was set at a p-value of <0.05.

3. Results

In total, 222 participants responded to the survey. A total of 54 responses were in paper form (24.3%), while the majority of responses were collected through the online version (75.7%, $n = 168$). The total number of participants consisted of participants who are still attending or have completed a postgraduate master's program in Pediatric and Preventive Dentistry in Germany, general dental practitioners in Germany, and members of the German Society for Pediatric Dentistry (DGKiZ e.V.). As efforts were made to invite as many practitioners as possible to participate in the survey, participants were asked to forward the online version of the questionnaire to colleagues in the same field. Thus, the precise number of participants who received the invitation and the exact response rate could not be calculated.

Table 1 shows the five cases of the questionnaire with the suggested scenarios and all the treatment options that were available in the questionnaire, as well as the percentages of the answers of the participants for each scenario (↑: cooperative child, ↓: uncooperative Child, P+: pain symptoms, P−: no pain symptoms) categorized into the three above-mentioned groups.

Table 2 provides the demographic and biographic characteristics of the respondents, along with the results of the negative binomial regression to investigate the variables' relation to the total number of not recommended/contraindicated treatment options for each participant.

The Pearson correlation and Mann–Whitney tests revealed no significant association between choosing the "not recommended/contraindicated" treatment options with any of the study variables, such as years of experience, the educational background of the dentist in pediatric dentistry, the number of patients per week, etc. (Table 2).

The total of answers in the not recommended category in the five cases ranged from 18.7 to 36.1% according to the cases, regardless of the specific scenarios, as illustrated in Figure 1. Case 4 (cavitated D2 approximal lesion) showed the highest percentage of chosen not recommended treatment options (36.1%), while case 1 (inactive lesions) had the lowest percentage with 18.7%. The differences between the cases in the distribution of answers to the assigned categories were statistically significant, as shown by the chi-square independent test ($p < 0.01$).

When considering the specific scenarios, regardless of the cases, there were statistically significant differences between the scenarios in the distribution of the answers, as depicted in Figure 2 (chi-square test $p < 0.01$). The percentages of the chosen not recommended treatment options for the scenarios "no pain and uncooperative patient" and "pain and cooperative patient" (32.6% and 31.0%, respectively) were higher than for the scenarios "no pain and cooperative patient" and "pain and uncooperative patient" (23.9% and 26.3% respectively).

Table 2. The demographic characteristics of the study population and the correlation of these variables with the number of not recommended/contraindicated answers.

	Mean Value ± SD	p-Value (Negative Binomial Regression as Continuous Variable)	Groups	Total Number	p-Value (Negative Binomial Regression as Categorial Variable)
Age	37.1 ± 9.8	0.582	-	-	-
Sex	-	-	Male	61 (27.5%)	0.704
			Female	161 (72.5%)	
Children treated per week	45.7 ± 78.2	0.402	-	-	-
Experience as a dentist (years)	11.7 ± 9.1	0.972	-	-	-
Experience with nitrous oxide sedation (years)	2.4 ± 4.9	0.403	Yes	104 (46.8%)	0.999
			No	118 (53.2%)	
Experience with GA (years)	4.89 ± 7.1	0.768	Yes	147 (66.2%)	0.534
			No	75 (33.8%)	
Experience as specialist pediatric dentist (years)	3.03 ± 5.3	0.649	Yes	120 (54.1%)	0.341
			No	102 (45.9%)	

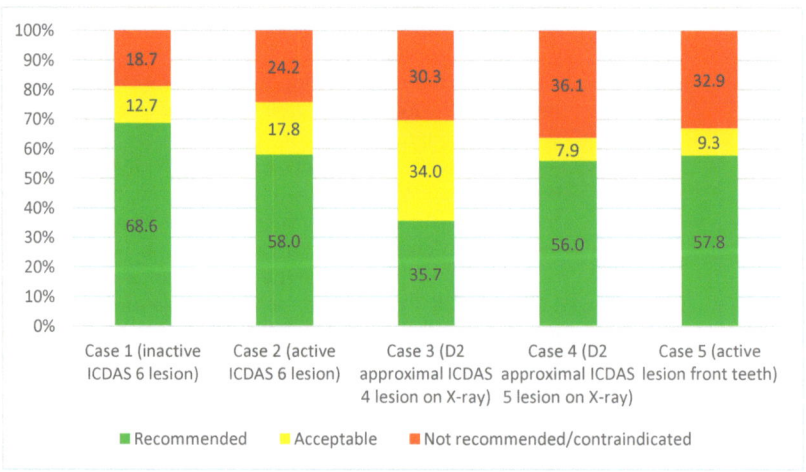

Figure 1. The percentages of the treatment options in the different cases were categorized according to the level of recommendation (n = 888 answers for each case in the four different scenarios from the 222 participants), differentiated by recommended, acceptable, and not recommended/contraindicated.

The percentage of the chosen not recommended/contraindicated treatment options did not differ when considering only the cooperation level of the child regardless of the pain symptoms. In contrast, the percentage of the chosen recommended treatment options was much less in scenarios with limited cooperation (Figure 3). These differences were statistically significant, as shown by the chi-square independent test ($p < 0.01$). The same pattern was also observed when considering pain symptoms regardless of the cooperation level, where pain symptoms lead to fewer chosen recommended treatment options (Figure 4). The differences between the scenarios "pain" and "no pain" in the distribution of answers to the assigned categories were statistically significant, as shown by the chi-square independent test ($p < 0.01$).

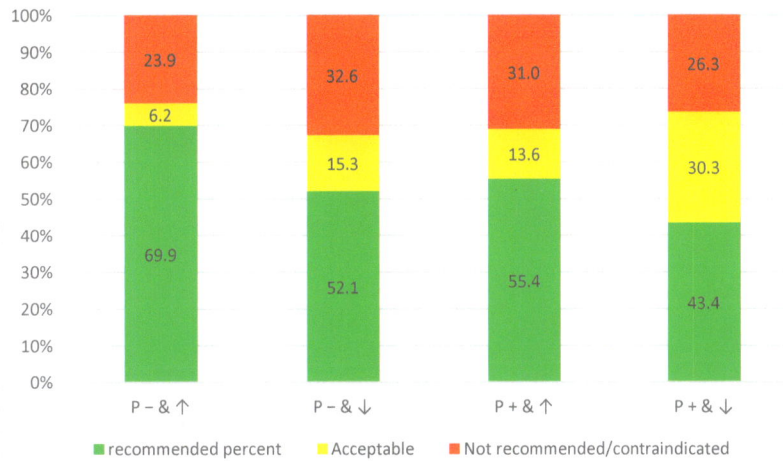

Figure 2. The categorization of the chosen treatment options regarding the suggested scenarios from the cases pooled together and shown as percentages (n = 888 answers for each scenario from all cases for the 222 participants). Differentiated by recommended, acceptable, and not recommended/contraindicated for ↑: cooperative child, ↓: uncooperative Child, P+: pain symptoms, and P−: no pain symptoms.

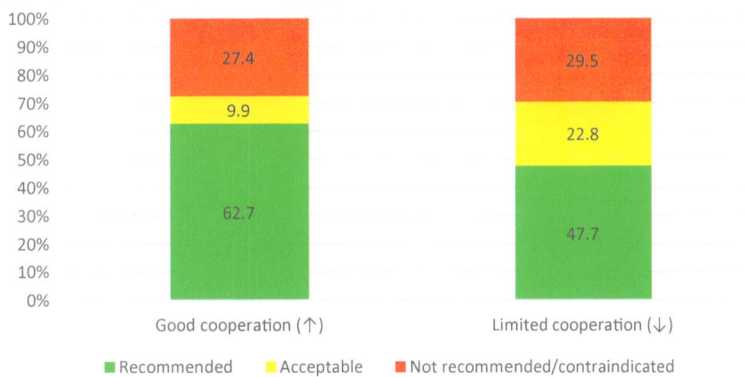

Figure 3. The categorization of the chosen treatment options regarding the cooperation of the patient from the cases pooled together, shown in percentages (n = 888 answers for each scenario from all cases for the 222 participants). ↑: cooperative child, ↓: uncooperative child.

Among the treatment options as seen in Table 1 that were classified in the category "not recommended and contraindicated" for specific scenarios, there were eight treatment options that were selected by more than 30% of the participants in these specific scenarios, which are further summarized and explained in Table 3.

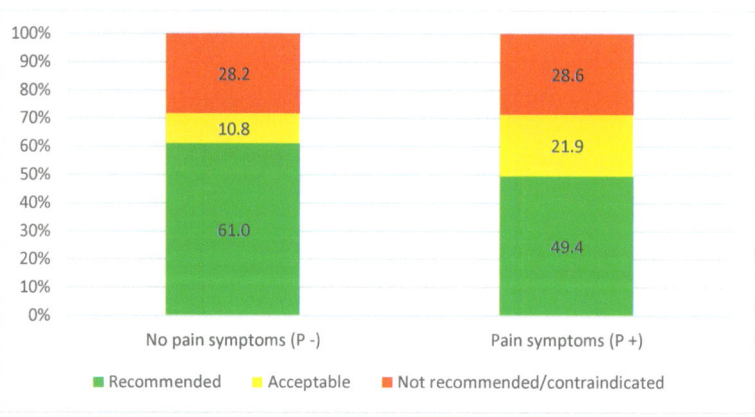

Figure 4. The categorization of the chosen treatment options regarding the symptoms of the patient from the cases pooled together, shown in percentages (n = 888 answers for each scenario from all cases for the 222 participants). P+: pain symptoms, P−: no pain symptoms.

Table 3. The treatment options, contraindicated or not recommended in specific scenarios, were chosen in ≥10% of these specific scenarios by participants, with the explanation for grouping them as contraindicated.

Treatment Option and Scenario	"Not Recommended/Contraindicated" Answers in %	Reason of Contraindication
Case 2 (Scenario: P− and ↑) Compomer filling (complete caries removal) in deep cavity	17.1%	Although symptomless, complete caries excavation in deep carious lesions is not recommended due to the risk of pulp exposure [13–15].
Case 2 (Scenario: P− and ↑) SSC in conventional technique (complete caries removal, preparation) in deep cavity	10.8%	Although symptomless, complete caries excavation in deep carious lesions is not recommended due to the risk of pulp exposure [13–15].
Case 3 (Scenario: P+ and ↓) Pulpotomy and SSC (caries media) under general anesthesia	20.3%	In this case, the pain was described as sensitivity on trigger, which indicates reversible pulpitis. GA carries risks of major and minor complications and should be avoided if possible [16,17]. There is no indication for GA as the carious lesion is not deep and, despite low cooperation, can be treated with minimal invasive options that do not require cooperation, such as the Hall technique [9,18].
Case 4 (Scenario: P− and ↑) Treatment of active caries approximal and occlusal ICDAS 4 with compomer filling (complete caries removal)	25.2%	Although symptomless, complete caries excavation in deep proximal carious lesions is not recommended due to the risk of pulp exposure [13–15].
Case 4 (Scenario: P− and ↓) Treatment of active caries approximal and occlusal ICDAS 4 with pulpotomy and SSC under general anesthesia	14.9%	GA carries risks of major and minor complications and should be avoided if possible [16,17]. There is no indication for GA as the carious lesion is not deep and, despite low cooperation, can be treated with minimal invasive options that do not require cooperation, such as the HT [9,18].

Table 3. Cont.

Treatment Option and Scenario	"Not Recommended/Contraindicated" Answers in %	Reason of Contraindication
Case 5 (Scenario: P− and ↓) EEC in a 3-year-old with primary maxillary anterior teeth with active caries, extraction under general anesthesia	11.3%	GA carries risks of major and minor complications and should be avoided if possible [16,17]. There is no indication for GA as the carious lesion is not deep and, despite low cooperation, can be treated with minimal invasive options that do not require cooperation, such as the SDF [9].
Case 5 (Scenario: P+ and ↑) EEC in a 3-year-old with primary maxillary anterior teeth with active caries, extraction of the front primary teeth under general anesthesia	17.1%	GA carries risks of major and minor complications and should be avoided if possible [16]. There is no indication for GA as the child is cooperative and treatment may be performed with local anesthesia and behavioral management techniques [19].
Case 5 (Scenario: P+ and ↑) EEC in a 3-year-old with primary maxillary anterior teeth with active caries, strip crown composite restorations	10.4%	Pain without stimulus is a symptom of irreversible pulpitis, where the teeth should not be filled without a pulpotomy/pulpectomy [20].

4. Discussion

This study aimed to explore and analyze decision-making processes among dental professionals in the field of pediatric dentistry. Understanding the methods employed and the characteristics of the study sample is crucial for interpreting the findings and assessing the generalizability of the results. To the authors' knowledge, this is the first research in Germany to explore dental decision-making in pediatric dentistry, which also includes various samples with different clinical backgrounds. The hypothetical clinical case scenarios can measure opinions about the care that might be provided in one particular case [21]. These scenarios and cases are not a tool for measuring the actual care a dentist would provide, as this will also be subjective to other factors that are not enclosed in a scenario, such as parental wishes, financial aspects, and the availability of treatment options in practice.

This study is a questionnaire-based survey focused on self-reporting. Such methods have gained more popularity in recent years in medical research [22], as they can give more understanding of real-life clinical daily practice. In order to recruit as many participants as possible, the questionnaire was available in both paper-based and online formats, which allowed for a varied participant pool, considering the varying preferences and convenience of potential respondents [23]. The total number of respondents ($n = 222$) offers a generous dataset for analyzing decision-making trends in pediatric dentistry, where the majority of respondents are females, reflecting the gender distribution among young dentists in Germany [24], especially in pediatric dentistry, with the majority of the members of the DGKiZ e.V. being females [25]. A deeper look at the demographic background of the study population shows different backgrounds regarding the years and places of undergraduate dental education. This means that the base of dental knowledge of the participants is from different schools and concepts, which might lead to variability in decision-making [26]. A great variety was observed in all the other demographic characteristics of the study population, such as years of experience and the number of children treated per week, etc. This variety enriches the study's external validity, capturing a range of perspectives from individuals at different stages of their dental careers, which makes the study population as near as possible to the real-life situation of practicing dental professionals, in order to be more representative of the target group as recommended in such surveys [27]. The study population's variety and heterogenicity were reflected in the experience in sedation techniques in pediatric dentistry, where 66.2% of the respondents had experience with GA compared to only 46.8% with experience in nitrous oxide. This might be the reason behind many participants also choosing invasive GA in cases of good cooperation to treat acute pain and in cases of no cooperation and no pain symptoms instead of choosing less invasive treatment options, probably with the aid of nitrous oxide sedation, which could reduce the need for dental GA in children [28]. A possible explanation for the higher number of participants with experience in GA compared to nitrous oxide is the fact that the National Health Insurance in Germany would cover the costs of GA sedation if justified by a lack of cooperation and the presence of dental treatment need for children under the age of 12 [29], while the patient would individually cover the costs of nitrous oxide sedation.

Overall, most of the answers in all cases with different scenarios were within the recommended and acceptable treatment spectrum. Still, seven out of the twenty scenarios of the cases had a total of not recommended or contraindicated treatment options of more than 30%. Three of these seven cases were cases 3, 4, and 5 with a scenario of lack of cooperation and no pain symptoms, where the dentists tend to recommend the GA. However, the caries could be inactivated and arrested, with a great chance of healing the pulp due to the absence of pain symptoms. The case with the highest percentage of not recommended and contraindicated answers (61.3%) was the case of Early Childhood Caries with pain symptoms and good cooperation, where the recommendation should be towards teeth extraction or endodontical treatment, probably chairside or under nitrous oxide sedation, rather than fillings or strip crowns under GA. This might reflect the pressure to achieve esthetics in the area of anterior teeth in young children, as parents are more willing to accept non-esthetic treatment options for their children in posterior teeth than in the upper anterior teeth [30]. Besides the treatment modality, the choice of the restoration type was in many of the cases towards dental fillings, either using compomer or composites, which is similar to another questionnaire study in Saudi Arabia where 73.8% of the dentists also reported the use of composite fillings on carious primary teeth [31]. However, there are clear recommendations to use prefabricated crowns rather than fillings, especially in multi-surfaced lesions in primary molars [9,13,32], due to the clear, better longevity of the crowns, with less failure over a longer period of time [6].

As our results clearly show, pain symptoms and the cooperation of the child greatly influence the treatment options and recommendations of the dentists, potentially leading to choices that may not align with the guidelines and recommendations. In our results, the scenarios with limited cooperation clearly had a higher percentage of not recommended answers and a lower percentage of recommended answers, highlighting the influence of the cooperation level of the child on the decision-making process. While the lack of cooperation is mostly linked to dental fear, a study in Japan was able to prove that cooperation and dental fear do not have a causal relationship [33], necessitating the need for behavioral management concepts and techniques in pediatric dentistry to avoid the need to treat every uncooperative child under GA [1]. Signs of dental fear and anxiety can be predicted at the very first appointment [34], resulting in planning suitable steps for stepwise treatments, which in turn can prevent the failure of treatment due to a lack of cooperation. Almost analogous to the influence of cooperation levels, the presence of pain symptoms resulted in fewer recommended answers, showing also an influence on decision-making. However, it must be noted that pain response is individualized and influenced by various factors inherent to the procedural context [35]. Moreover, child-reported pain symptoms, especially in small children, are not valid and clearly defined. In our study, we used the terms "pain", "spontaneous pain", and "sensitivity", which are descriptive of different states of clinical situations resulting in a different diagnosis. It cannot be excluded that the participants of this study did not quite differentiate between these terms, which would influence the decision-making process, as many practitioners in pediatric dentistry might not put a value on the patient-reported symptoms and concentrate mainly on clinical and radiographical examinations to reach their decisions, due to the limitations of self-reporting in children. However, pain and cooperation do influence each other, as sudden pain during treatments in children might cause a lack of cooperation in future sessions [36]. The dentists are, therefore, encouraged to minimize the experience of pain and discomfort during pediatric dental treatment, e.g., with the administration of local anesthesia [35,37]. The elimination of procedural pain would allow for a better judgment of symptomatic pain of dental origin.

Considering the differences between the cases regardless of the different suggested scenarios, it was observed that case 4, showing a deep ICDAS 5 approximal carious lesion on a primary molar, had the highest percentage of not recommended or contraindicated answers (32.9%). In contrast, case 3, showing an ICDAS 4 approximal carious lesion on a primary molar, had the lowest percentage of recommended answers (35.7%). This reflects the great challenges and difficulties practitioners face in diagnosing and treating approximal carious lesions in children and highlights the need for further education and training in this area. Restorative treatment thresholds based on radiographic lesion depth also vary substantially among dentists on permanent teeth in adults [38], where the problems of cooperation and pain are not relevant, as in pediatric patients. Our results could not detect true patterns or risk factors leading to an increased number of not recommended or contraindicated answers on an individual level, which might be due to the great heterogenicity of the study population. However, this heterogenicity reflects the actual diversity among practitioners actively practicing pediatric dentistry. Therefore, it cannot be concluded that more experienced dentists make better decisions or that younger practitioners are aware of the actual recommendations. Dental practitioners are thus encouraged to always seek further education to keep up-to-date with the latest updates and recommendations based on recent studies.

Our results showed a great variation in decision-making among pediatric dentists, which may be due to several factors. The most obvious explanation could be the great variations in the study population's educational/clinical background [26] and work experience [39]. The differences and variations in decision-making should not be considered disadvantageous in general, as it is also noticeable in other dental specialties such as restorative dentistry [40]. Most commonly, dentists gain most of their knowledge in their undergraduate studies and adopt treatment scenarios and experiences of their own through the years, which become very challenging to change over time due to multiple barriers, such as the lack of knowledge and fear of making mistakes [41,42]. However, when it comes to making decisions for treatments using sedation techniques that carry high risks of complications such as GA [17], clinicians must be well aware of other alternatives such as nitrous oxide sedation and the possibility of non- or minimally invasive management options for dental caries when no pulpal involvement (such as indicated by pain symptoms) is clear, even with limited cooperation due to very young age. Nevertheless, these results should be interpreted with caution, as decision-making is a very complex process where many factors play a role and interact with each other, and due to the difficulties defining a gold standard with "correct" and "wrong" answers. In the planning of this study, efforts were made to build a categorization that would represent the most up-to-date recommendations and guidelines and to include the aspect of clinical experience through a team of multiple experienced specialized pediatric dentists with leading roles in teaching pediatric dentistry on the national and international levels. To minimize bias in the assessments of the answers, the treatment options for each case and scenario were categorized before the data analysis and are shown transparently in Table 1.

As in any other research, our study has several limitations that should be considered when interpreting the results. Most important is the generalizability and representativity of the study sample. Although the data collection process considered all potential practicing pediatric dentists, this specialty in Germany is not exclusively for specialists and could be practiced by general practitioners. Although all the members of the DGKiZ listed on their website were contacted ($n = 360$), only 11.4% ($n = 41$) of them responded by completing the survey. Moreover, the total number of DGKiZ members is nearly 1900, meaning the members listed on the website represent less than 20% of the members. Therefore, our results can give an idea about the variation and differences in decision-making among a sample of practicing pediatric dentists but does not represent all pediatric dentists in Germany. Another limitation of the study is the design of the questions on the tooth level, with the consideration of pain and cooperation on the patient level, while the real-life approach would have been to design the questions showing the whole dentition and adding questions regarding every tooth, to make more realistic decisions, especially considering GA. On the other hand, designing the questionnaire in this manner would lengthen the questionnaire and probably decrease the response rate dramatically, making the analysis and the results even more complex. Nevertheless, this study also has strengths that need to be discussed; the inclusion of pain and cooperation in such a questionnaire is an addition to many similar studies, and it showed a great influence on the decision-making. Moreover, the heterogenicity of the study population gives a closer look into the variety of the community in general and especially among practicing dentists, including experienced as well as freshly graduated dentists, who are either committed to pediatric dentistry and treat more patients per week or who only partially treat children, besides performing regular dental treatments on adults.

5. Conclusions

A great variety in dental decision-making was observed among practicing pediatric dentists in Germany. Pain symptoms and cooperation levels influence the decisions of the practitioner, with an especial risk of too invasive treatment options in low-severity cases. A notable portion of the practitioners may suggest treatment options that might be considered not recommended or even contraindicated, highlighting the need for adhering to evidence-based dental guidelines and recommendations in daily practice and the need for continuous education over the years.

Author Contributions: Conceptualization, B.A.R. and J.S.; methodology, B.A.R., J.S. and A.A.M.; formal analysis, B.A.R. and A.A.M.; investigation, B.A.R. and J.S.; writing—original draft preparation, B.A.R., M.A. and A.A.M.; writing—review and editing, A.A.M., J.S. and C.H.S.; supervision, J.S. and C.H.S.; All authors have read and agreed to the published version of the manuscript.

Funding: This research received no external funding.

Institutional Review Board Statement: Ethical Committee of the University of Greifswald BB 052/20 "Dental Decision Taking" in dentists in pediatric dentistry, approved on 2 April 2020.

Informed Consent Statement: Informed consent was obtained from all subjects involved in the study to analyze the data and publish the results.

Data Availability Statement: The original contributions presented in this study are included in the article. Further inquiries can be directed to the corresponding author.

Conflicts of Interest: The authors declare no conflicts of interest.

References

1. Klinberg, G. Dental anxiety and behaviour management problems in paediatric dentistry—A review of background factors and diagnostics. *Eur. Arch. Paediatr. Dent.* **2008**, *9* (Suppl. S1), 11–15. [CrossRef] [PubMed]
2. Schwendicke, F.; Krois, J.; Splieth, C.H.; Innes, N.; Robertson, M.; Schmoeckel, J.; Santamaria, R.M. Cost-effectiveness of managing cavitated primary molar caries lesions: A randomized trial in Germany. *J. Dent.* **2018**, *78*, 40–45. [CrossRef]
3. Splieth, C.H.; Banerjee, A.; Bottenberg, P.; Breschi, L.; Campus, G.; Ekstrand, K.R.; Giacaman, R.A.; Haak, R.; Hannig, M.; Hickel, R.; et al. How to Intervene in the Caries Process in Children: A Joint ORCA and EFCD Expert Delphi Consensus Statement. *Caries Res.* **2020**, *54*, 297–305. [CrossRef] [PubMed]
4. Finkeissen, E. *Dental Decision Making, A Foundation for Knowledge-Based Second Opinions*; Finkeissen, E., Ed.; Die Deutsche Bibliothek—CIP-Einzelaufnahme: Heidelberg, Germany, 2002. Available online: https://www.klinikum.uni-heidelberg.de/fileadmin/inst_med_biometrie/med_Informatik/pdf/DentDecMak_EF.pdf (accessed on 17 November 2024).
5. Amend, S.; Boutsiouki, C.; Bekes, K.; Kloukos, D.; Lygidakis, N.N.; Frankenberger, R.; Kramer, N. Clinical effectiveness of restorative materials for the restoration of carious primary teeth without pulp therapy: A systematic review. *Eur. Arch. Paediatr. Dent.* **2022**, *23*, 727–759. [CrossRef] [PubMed]
6. Potter, L.A.; Vollmer, M.; Santamaria, R.M.; Splieth, C.H.; Schmoeckel, J. Performance of restorations in primary molars over a seven-year period. *J. Dent.* **2024**, *147*, 105121. [CrossRef]

7. Elhennawy, K.; Finke, C.; Paris, S.; Reda, S.; Jost-Brinkmann, P.G.; Schwendicke, F. Selective vs stepwise removal of deep carious lesions in primary molars: 24 months follow-up from a randomized controlled trial. *Clin. Oral Investig.* **2021**, *25*, 645–652. [CrossRef]
8. Innes, N.P.; Evans, D.J.; Stirrups, D.R. Sealing caries in primary molars: Randomized control trial, 5-year results. *J. Dent. Res.* **2011**, *90*, 1405–1410. [CrossRef]
9. BaniHani, A.; Santamaria, R.M.; Hu, S.; Maden, M.; Albadri, S. Minimal intervention dentistry for managing carious lesions into dentine in primary teeth: An umbrella review. *Eur. Arch. Paediatr. Dent.* **2022**, *23*, 667–693. [CrossRef]
10. Innes, N.P.; Evans, D.J.; Stirrups, D.R. The Hall Technique; a randomized controlled clinical trial of a novel method of managing carious primary molars in general dental practice: Acceptability of the technique and outcomes at 23 months. *BMC Oral Health* **2007**, *7*, 18. [CrossRef]
11. Zaffarano, L.; Salerno, C.; Campus, G.; Cirio, S.; Balian, A.; Karanxha, L.; Cagetti, M.G. Silver Diamine Fluoride (SDF) Efficacy in Arresting Cavitated Caries Lesions in Primary Molars: A Systematic Review and Metanalysis. *Int. J. Environ. Res. Public Health* **2022**, *19*, 12917. [CrossRef]
12. Hu, S.; BaniHani, A.; Nevitt, S.; Maden, M.; Santamaria, R.M.; Albadri, S. Hall technique for primary teeth: A systematic review and meta-analysis. *Jpn. Dent. Sci. Rev.* **2022**, *58*, 286–297. [CrossRef] [PubMed]
13. Tedesco, T.K.; Reis, T.M.; Mello-Moura, A.C.V.; Silva, G.S.D.; Scarpini, S.; Floriano, I.; Gimenez, T.; Mendes, F.M.; Raggio, D.P. Management of deep caries lesions with or without pulp involvement in primary teeth: A systematic review and network meta-analysis. *Braz. Oral Res.* **2020**, *35*, e004. [CrossRef] [PubMed]
14. Aiem, E.; Joseph, C.; Garcia, A.; Smail-Faugeron, V.; Muller-Bolla, M. Caries removal strategies for deep carious lesions in primary teeth: Systematic review. *Int. J. Paediatr. Dent.* **2020**, *30*, 392–404. [CrossRef] [PubMed]
15. Duggal, M.; Gizani, S.; Albadri, S.; Kramer, N.; Stratigaki, E.; Tong, H.J.; Seremidi, K.; Kloukos, D.; BaniHani, A.; Santamaria, R.M.; et al. Best clinical practice guidance for treating deep carious lesions in primary teeth: An EAPD policy document. *Eur. Arch. Paediatr. Dent.* **2022**, *23*, 659–666. [CrossRef]
16. Mortazavi, H.; Baharvand, M.; Safi, Y. Death Rate of Dental Anaesthesia. *J. Clin. Diagn. Res.* **2017**, *11*, ZE07–ZE09. [CrossRef]
17. Erkmen Almaz, M.; Akbay Oba, A.; Saroglu Sonmez, I. Postoperative morbidity in pediatric patients following dental treatment under general anesthesia. *Eur. Oral Res.* **2019**, *53*, 113–118. [CrossRef]
18. Badar, S.B.; Tabassum, S.; Khan, F.R.; Ghafoor, R. Effectiveness of Hall Technique for Primary Carious Molars: A Systematic Review and Meta-analysis. *Int. J. Clin. Pediatr. Dent.* **2019**, *12*, 445–452. [CrossRef]
19. Peedikayil, F.C.; Vijayan, A. An update on local anesthesia for pediatric dental patients. *Anesth. Essays Res.* **2013**, *7*, 4–9. [CrossRef] [PubMed]
20. Wolters, W.J.; Duncan, H.F.; Tomson, P.L.; Karim, I.E.; McKenna, G.; Dorri, M.; Stangvaltaite, L.; van der Sluis, L.W.M. Minimally invasive endodontics: A new diagnostic system for assessing pulpitis and subsequent treatment needs. *Int. Endod. J.* **2017**, *50*, 825–829. [CrossRef]
21. Kateeb, E.T.; Warren, J.J.; Gaeth, G.J.; Momany, E.T.; Damiano, P.C. Understanding Pediatric Dentists' Dental Caries Management Treatment Decisions: A Conjoint Experiment. *JDR Clin. Trans. Res.* **2016**, *1*, 86–94. [CrossRef]
22. Duffett, M.; Burns, K.E.; Adhikari, N.K.; Arnold, D.M.; Lauzier, F.; Kho, M.E.; Meade, M.O.; Hayani, O.; Koo, K.; Choong, K.; et al. Quality of reporting of surveys in critical care journals: A methodologic review. *Crit. Care Med.* **2012**, *40*, 441–449. [CrossRef] [PubMed]
23. Uhlig, C.E.; Seitz, B.; Eter, N.; Promesberger, J.; Busse, H. Efficiencies of Internet-based digital and paper-based scientific surveys and the estimated costs and time for different-sized cohorts. *PLoS ONE* **2014**, *9*, e108441. [CrossRef] [PubMed]
24. Bundeszahnärztekammer. Statistical Yearbook of the German Federal Dental Association. Available online: https://www.bzaek.de/ueber-uns/daten-und-zahlen/nachgezaehlt.html (accessed on 7 October 2024).
25. DGKiZ. News from the German Society for Pediatric Dentistry. *Oralprophylaxe Kinderzahnheilkd.* **2020**, *42*, 118–119.
26. Marinho, V.C.; Richards, D.; Niederman, R. Variation, certainty, evidence, and change in dental education: Employing evidence-based dentistry in dental education. *J. Dent. Educ.* **2001**, *65*, 449–455. [CrossRef] [PubMed]
27. Fincham, J.E. Response rates and responsiveness for surveys, standards, and the Journal. *Am. J. Pharm. Educ.* **2008**, *72*, 43. [CrossRef] [PubMed]
28. Mourad, M.S.; Splieth, C.H.; Al Masri, A.; Schmoeckel, J. Potential for nitrous oxide sedation in pedodontics practice to reduce the need for dental general anesthesia. *Quintessence Int.* **2022**, *53*, 598–606. [CrossRef]
29. Kassenzahnärztliche Bundesvereinigung. [General Anesthesia at the Dentist—When Does the Health Insurance Pay?] Available online: https://www.kzbv.de/kzbv2021-pi-vollnarkose.download.68527610c984873a13996098757c79f3.pdf (accessed on 7 October 2024). (In German)
30. Sabbagh, H.; Othman, M.; Khogeer, L.; Al-Harbi, H.; Al Harthi, A.; Abdulgader Yaseen Abdulgader, A. Parental acceptance of silver Diamine fluoride application on primary dentition: A systematic review and meta-analysis. *BMC Oral Health* **2020**, *20*, 227. [CrossRef]
31. Halawany, H.S.; Salama, F.; Jacob, V.; Abraham, N.B.; Moharib, T.N.B.; Alazmah, A.S.; Al Harbi, J.A. A survey of pediatric dentists' caries-related treatment decisions and restorative modalities—A web-based survey. *Saudi Dent. J.* **2017**, *29*, 66–73. [CrossRef]
32. Santamaria, R.M.; Abudrya, M.H.; Gul, G.; Mourad, M.S.; Gomez, G.F.; Zandona, A.G.F. How to Intervene in the Caries Process: Dentin Caries in Primary Teeth. *Caries Res.* **2020**, *54*, 306–323. [CrossRef]

33. Yamada, M.K.; Tanabe, Y.; Sano, T.; Noda, T. Cooperation during dental treatment: The Children's Fear Survey Schedule in Japanese children. *Int. J. Paediatr. Dent.* **2002**, *12*, 404–409. [CrossRef]
34. Klaassen, M.; Veerkamp, J.; Hoogstraten, J. Predicting dental anxiety. The clinical value of anxiety questionnaires: An explorative study. *Eur. J. Paediatr. Dent.* **2003**, *4*, 171–176. [PubMed]
35. Young, K.D. Pediatric procedural pain. *Ann. Emerg. Med.* **2005**, *45*, 160–171. [CrossRef] [PubMed]
36. Milsom, K.M.; Tickle, M.; Humphris, G.M.; Blinkhorn, A.S. The relationship between anxiety and dental treatment experience in 5-year-old children. *Br. Dent. J.* **2003**, *194*, 503–506; discussion 495. [CrossRef]
37. Ghanei, M.; Arnrup, K.; Robertson, A. Procedural pain in routine dental care for children: A part of the Swedish BITA study. *Eur. Arch. Paediatr. Dent.* **2018**, *19*, 365–372. [CrossRef]
38. Gordan, V.V.; Garvan, C.W.; Richman, J.S.; Fellows, J.L.; Rindal, D.B.; Qvist, V.; Heft, M.W.; Williams, O.D.; Gilbert, G.H.; Group, D.C. How dentists diagnose and treat defective restorations: Evidence from the dental practice-based research network. *Oper. Dent.* **2009**, *34*, 664–673. [CrossRef] [PubMed]
39. Qudeimat, M.A.; Al-Saiegh, F.A.; Al-Omari, Q.; Omar, R. Restorative treatment decisions for deep proximal carious lesions in primary molars. *Eur. Arch. Paediatr. Dent.* **2007**, *8*, 37–42. [CrossRef]
40. Kay, E.J.; Locker, D. Variations in restorative treatment decisions: An international comparison. *Community Dent. Oral Epidemiol.* **1996**, *24*, 376–379. [CrossRef]
41. Innes, N.P.; Frencken, J.E.; Schwendicke, F. Don't Know, Can't Do, Won't Change: Barriers to Moving Knowledge to Action in Managing the Carious Lesion. *J. Dent. Res.* **2016**, *95*, 485–486. [CrossRef]
42. Jeggle, L.M.; Baker, S.R.; Schwendicke, F. Changing dentists' carious tissue removal behavior: Qualitative study and behavioral change simulation experiment. *J. Dent.* **2019**, *81*, 43–51. [CrossRef]

Disclaimer/Publisher's Note: The statements, opinions and data contained in all publications are solely those of the individual author(s) and contributor(s) and not of MDPI and/or the editor(s). MDPI and/or the editor(s) disclaim responsibility for any injury to people or property resulting from any ideas, methods, instructions or products referred to in the content.

Article

Survival Analysis of Glass Ionomer Cement and Resin-Based Sealant Retention: A 10-Year Follow-Up Study

Sandra Petrauskienė, Kristina Saldūnaitė-Mikučionienė and Julija Narbutaitė *

Department of Preventive and Paediatric Dentistry, Faculty of Odontology, Lithuanian University of Health Sciences, Luksos-Daumanto Str. 6, LT-50106 Kaunas, Lithuania; sandra.petrauskiene@lsmu.lt (S.P.); kristina.saldunaite@lsmu.lt (K.S.-M.)
* Correspondence: julija.narbutaite@lsmu.lt

Abstract: *Background and Objective*: Sealant application is a proven method to prevent occlusal caries; however, long-term studies on this topic are scarce. This study aimed to assess the survival rate and clinical effectiveness of glass ionomer cement (GIC) and resin-based sealants (RBSs) on second permanent molars over a long-term follow-up period. *Materials and methods:* Sixteen patients aged 11–13 years with all four completely erupted permanent second molars were enrolled in the study. All patients attended 1-year and 3-year follow-ups; however, one participant did not respond after 10 years and was excluded from the final analyses. The oral health status evaluation was based on WHO criteria. A total of 32 teeth received an RBS (Clinpro), and a further 32 teeth were sealed with GIC (Fuji IX). The sealant retention was determined according to the Kilpatrick criteria after 1 year, 3 years, and 10 years, respectively. Statistical analysis included a chi-square test, the Kaplan–Meier method, and the Cox proportional hazard model. *Results*: At baseline, seven boys and eight girls participated in the study, with a mean age of 12.3 ± 0.9 years. The 1-year follow-up results revealed that 90% of the RBSs and 43.3% of the GIC sealants were completely retained, and no caries lesions were recorded ($p = 0.01$). The 3-year follow-up results showed that 23.3% of the RBSs and 0% of the GIC sealants demonstrated complete retention ($p = 0.034$). Moreover, 10.0% of the occlusal surfaces in the RBS group and 13.3% of the occlusal surfaces in the GIC group were filled ($p > 0.05$). A total of 6.7% of the RBSs showed complete retention. One-third of the sealed teeth (30.0% of the teeth sealed with RBSs and 36.7% of teeth applied with GIC) were filled after 10 years. The Kaplan–Meier analysis demonstrated a higher survival rate in the RBS group when compared with the GIC over the entire follow-up period ($p = 0.001$). *Conclusions*: Although the survival rate of RBSs was higher than GIC sealants, their effectiveness in preventing fissure caries in permanent second molars did not differ significantly over a 10-year follow-up.

Keywords: caries prevention; resin-based sealant; glass ionomer sealant; fissure sealant; sealant retention

1. Introduction

Dental caries prevails as a chronic non-communicable disease in both children and adults, and it also remains the most relevant global oral health burden worldwide [1,2].

Caries prevention remains a challenge due to the high prevalence of disease in recently erupted teeth [3]. Early sealant application after permanent molar eruption allows one to achieve a higher effectiveness in caries prevention [4]. Handelman was the pioneer in terms of analyzing the role of sealant application over incipient dental caries lesions [5]. Studies have shown that teeth to which sealants have been applied may require less extensive dental treatment than teeth without sealants. Furthermore, patients with sealed teeth need less frequent restorative treatment in the future [6]. A systematic review revealed that the application of dental sealants may reduce caries development in permanent posterior teeth from 40% to 6% during a 2-year period [7].

The main indication for dental sealant application is recently erupted permanent teeth with deep pits and fissures [8]. The occlusal surfaces of molars tend to accumulate dental plaque because of pits and fissures, and these may play a role in the inefficient management of occlusal caries [9,10]. Thus, dental sealants are defined as an effective preventive procedure due to serving as a micromechanically bonded protective layer [9–11]. Pit and fissure sealants are applied not only for prevention but also for the management of incipient non-cavitated occlusal caries lesions.

The term "pit and fissure sealant" describes a chemically active liquid material that is applied to the occlusal pits and fissures of caries-susceptible teeth. Moreover, it is cured chemically or via light [6]. Pit and fissure sealants were introduced by Buonocore, who presented the acid etching technique and application procedure of pits and fissures to prevent caries in 1955 [12]. Glass ionomer cement (GIC) as a pit and fissure sealant was introduced by McLean and Wilson in 1974 [13].

When considering the chemical composition, there are two main categories of material, including resin-based sealants (RBSs) and glass ionomer cement (GIC). The most common subgroups of sealants, such as polyacid-modified resin sealants, resin-based sealants, resin-modified glass-ionomer sealants, and glass-ionomer sealants, have been evaluated in various studies [14]. Even flowable composites can be used as dental sealants [15]. However, resin-based sealants are defined as the gold standard [16]. A meta-analysis by Lam et al., 2021 proved that RBS application on permanent molars correlates with a reduction in occlusal caries development and with the arrest of caries lesion progression [17]. However, a significant disadvantage of resin-based sealants is their sensitivity to moisture during application procedures [10].

Glass ionomer cement as a dental sealant possesses certain advantages. Glass ionomer cement is a moisture-friendly dental material, and it is capable of releasing fluoride [10,18]. The technique of GIC application is easier to perform when compared to the application of resin-based sealants [19]. GIC enables one to ensure a potential preventive effect of fluoride release even after a high loss of sealed material [19,20]. Thus, this material is an option for partially erupted teeth [19,20]. In considering microleakages, certain brands, such as Fuji IX, are preferred over other GIC sealants [21]. The main drawback of GIC is its relatively poor retention [16,20]. However, it is acceptable to use GIC as a sealant in caries prevention programs [22].

The retention rate of sealants on tooth surfaces is the main indicator of their success [23].

The complete retention of pit and fissure sealants ensures optimal protection [16]. Meanwhile, the sites of dental plaque retention that are caused by the partial loss of sealant may initiate caries development [24]. Early pit and fissure sealant loss is related to salivary contamination during application procedures [25], and it is also dependent on the type of sealant material used [26]. Long-lasting caries prevention is aided by regular dental appointments and the resealing of susceptible tooth surfaces if the previously applied material is deficient [11,27].

Dental sealant is an integrated component of various prevention programs, such as non-operative caries treatment programs (e.g., the Nexö method) [28–30]. Subsequently, DMF-S was significantly reduced in the communities that implemented these programs [29,30]. In Lithuania, only 23.61% of schoolchildren have caries-free dentition [31]. The prevalence of caries in permanent molars was 41% among 5- to 6-year-olds [32] and 64.0% among 12-year-old school children in Lithuania [33]. The prevalence of dental caries among 12-year-olds has remained high (88.4% in 1983, 85.5% in 2005, and 70.6% in 2009) over the decades [33,34]. The mean DMF-T score was found to be high (7.9) among 12-year-old Lithuanian children [35]. This situation indicates a high (dental) treatment need, especially non-operative treatments, to control and reduce caries development in Lithuania [32,35].

The sealing of caries-free teeth or enamel-incipient lesions is recommended for patients who are at risk [25,29]. A national program of pit and fissure sealants was initiated in 2004 in Lithuania [36]. The target group for sealant application is children aged 5–13 years with recently erupted permanent molars. Saldūnaitė et al. found that 12-year-old Lithuanian children who had up to two teeth had pit and fissure sealants applied [33].

In considering the effectiveness of occlusal caries prevention, numerous studies have not defined the significant differences between resin-based sealants and glass ionomer cement ones [9].

This study aimed to assess the survival rate and clinical effectiveness of glass ionomer cement (GIC) and resin-based sealants (RBSs) on second permanent molars over a long-term follow-up period.

2. Materials and Methods

We conducted this clinical study of sealant retention in permanent second molars at the Clinic of Preventive and Pediatric Dentistry of the Lithuanian University of Health Sciences (LSMU) (Kaunas, Lithuania) during 2004–2016. The study was conducted in line with the principles of the Declaration of Helsinki. The Kaunas Regional Biomedical Research Ethics Committee approved the study protocol (no. 100/2003). The parents of the participants provided their written informed consent for the patients to participate in the study.

2.1. Participants

The study targeted patients aged 11–13 years who were attending the Clinic of Preventive and Pediatric Dentistry, LSMU in Kaunas, Lithuania. A total of 16 patients with all four fully erupted permanent second molars were enrolled in the study. The enrollment of participants was carried out from March 2004 until November 2005. Sealant application was performed between April 2004 and December 2005.

All patients attended 1-year and 3-year follow-ups, but one participant did not respond after 10 years and was thus excluded from the final analyses (Figure 1).

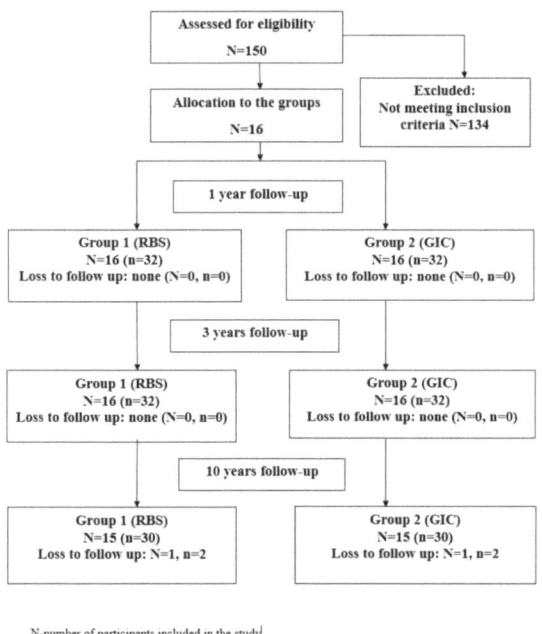

Figure 1. Flowchart diagram of the study sample.

2.1.1. Inclusion Criteria

The patient inclusion criteria were the following: 11–13-year-old patients without any known systemic diseases.

The teeth-related inclusion criteria were the following: maxillary and mandibular second permanent molars have completely erupted with sound and intact pits and fissures.

2.1.2. Exclusion Criteria

The patient exclusion criteria were the following: uncooperative patients and patients with mental and/or physical disorders.

The teeth-related exclusion criteria were the following: partially erupted second permanent molars, second permanent molars with proximal caries, and enamel with developmental defects, restorations, or sealants.

2.2. Sample Size Calculation

The sample size for the study was calculated using Power Analysis (G-power software™ (Release 3.0) Heinrich Heine University, Düsseldorf, Germany, for Windows). The sample size calculation provided a value of 16 participants (32 teeth per group) with a confidence level of 95% and a type I error (alpha) of 5% when a difference of 43.5% between the complete retention rates of the tested RBS and GIC was assumed at 12 months. A power of 98% indicated that the sample size of 16 participants (32 teeth per group) was sufficient.

2.3. Intervention

Prior to the sealant application, clinical examinations were performed and bitewing radiographs were taken to ensure that no caries lesions were present.

The oral health status evaluation was based on WHO criteria [37] under standardized conditions with a plane dental mirror and periodontal (CPI) probe in a dental clinic setting. During follow-ups, oral examinations were performed using the same criteria as the baseline visit. After a dental examination, the scores of the decayed, missed, and filled permanent teeth (DMF-T) index were calculated [38,39].

The presence of dental plaque in each participant was assessed using the Silness–Löe plaque index (PI). Dental plaque was recorded at the gingival areas of the buccal, mesial, distal, and palatal/lingual surfaces of all the teeth. The score for a tooth was counted by adding the scores of each area and dividing by 4. Meanwhile, the score for each patient was counted by adding all the scores of the teeth and then dividing this by the number of teeth, with ratings of 0 to 3 (0—excellent; 0.1–0.9—good; 1.0–1.9—fair; and 2.0–3.0—poor) [38].

Oral examinations, sealant applications, and follow-ups were performed by the same dental hygienist (specialist) (K.S-M).

Overall, sealants were applied to 64 teeth. Resin-based sealants (RBSs) (Clinpro™ Sealant, 3M/ESPE, Saint Paul, MN, USA) were applied to a total of 32 teeth, and 32 teeth were sealed with glass ionomer cement (GIC) sealants (Fuji IX, -Fuji IX, GC, Tokyo, Japan) at baseline. The sealants were applied in accordance with the manufacturers' instructions (Figure 2). The material for sealant (RBS or GIC) application, with regard to the upper or lower jaw and side (right or left), was selected by the operator. Additionally, moisture control conditions were considered.

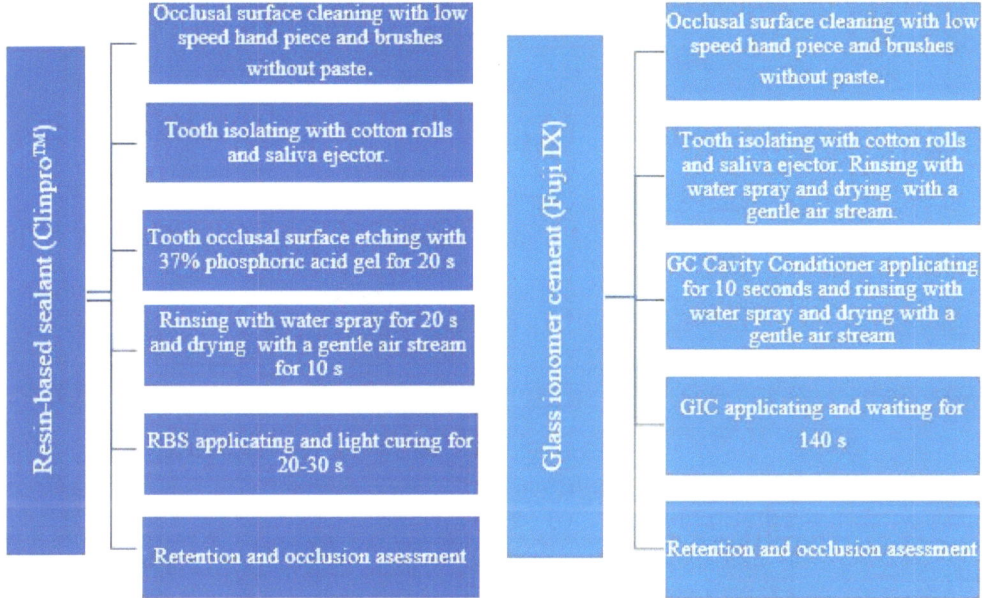

Figure 2. The step-by-step sealant application procedures for both materials (RBSs and GIC).

Professional oral hygiene was performed, and regular oral hygiene instructions were given to all participants at the beginning and during follow-up appointments.

2.4. Outcome Measurement

The integrity of the sealant was assessed clinically during the follow-up appointments after 1 year, 3 years, and 10 years of placement. The retention of the sealant material on each sealed tooth was determined according to the Kilpatrick criteria [40] as follows: 0 indicates complete retention, 1 indicates the loss of 1/3 of the sealant, 2 indicates the loss of 2/3 of the sealant, and 3 indicates the complete loss of the sealant (more than 2/3 of the material). The later scores of sealant retention were regrouped as complete retention (score 0), partial loss (scores 1 and 2), and total loss (score 3). In addition, all the surfaces of the teeth sealed with sealants were evaluated in terms of caries development during follow-up visits. The criteria for evaluation were the following: 0 indicates no caries, and 1 indicates caries (filling) present [41]. Later, "failure" was defined as a partial loss of the sealant or a complete loss of the sealed material and filling.

2.5. Statistical Analysis

A statistical analysis was performed using the Statistical Package for Social Sciences (SPSS version 29). A chi-square test served to measure the differences between the assessed sealant groups. The Mann–Whitney U test was used to compare the mean scores of the PI at different time periods. A comparison of different time periods with respect to the mean scores of the DMF-T index and its components (D-T, M-T, and F-T) was performed using the Wilcoxon test. A survival analysis of the different sealant materials was performed with the Kaplan–Meier method and the Cox proportional hazard model. The significance level was set at $p < 0.05$.

3. Results

Table 1 shows the demographic characteristics of the study participants, as follows: seven boys (46.7%) and eight girls (53.3%), with a mean age of 12.3 ± 0.9 years at the baseline.

Table 1. Characteristics of the participants by year and gender at the baseline.

	N	%
Age (N = 15)		
11 years	4	26.7
12 years	3	20.0
13 years	8	53.3
Total	15	100.0
MS ± SD (years)	12.3 ± 0.9	
Gender (N = 15)		
Boy (male)	7	46.7
Girl (female)	8	53.3
Total	15	100.0

MS ± SD—mean score ± standard deviation.

Table 2 shows the oral health status (presence of dental plaque (PI) and severity of dental caries (DMF-T)) of the study participants at the baseline and the 10-year follow-ups. At baseline, the mean score of the PI was 2.53 ± 0.50. The oral hygiene of the participants was slightly improved over the whole follow-up period, with a PI of 2.47 ± 0.62 ($p = 0.723$). Consequently, the mean score of the filled teeth (F-T) significantly increased during the 10-year follow-up period (from 0.93 ± 1.10 to 3.20 ± 2.43; $p = 0.013$). Within the same follow-up period, the dental caries severity (mean DMF-T score) had increased significantly (from 1.13 ± 1.25 to 3.60 ± 2.30; $p = 0.003$).

Table 2. Oral status of the participants over the whole follow-up period.

Variables	Follow-Up Period				p-Value
	Baseline MS ± SD	1-Year MS ± SD	3-Year MS ± SD	10-year MS ± SD	
Dental caries [a]					
D-T	0.20 ± 0.41	0.25 ± 0.12	0.31 ± 0.14	0.40 ± 1.30	1.00
M-T	0.0 ± 0.0	0.0 ± 0.0	0.0 ± 0.0	0.0 ± 0.0	1.00
F-T	0.93 ± 1.10 [b]	1.05 ± 0.19	1.4 ± 0.22	3.20 ± 2.43 [b]	0.013 [b]
DMF-T	1.13 ± 1.25 [b]	1.3 ± 1.15	1.71 ± 1.43	3.60 ± 2.30 [b]	0.003 [b]
Presence of dental plaque [c]					
PI	2.53 ± 0.50	2.73 ± 0.446 [b]	2.00 ± 0.638 [b]	2.47 ± 0.62	0.723 < 0.001 [b]

[a] Wilcoxon test. [b] significant difference between different follow-up periods. [c] Mann–Whitney U test. MS ± SD—mean score ± standard deviation.

At baseline, there were 32 permanent second molars sealed with RBSs and 32 sealed with GIC. Table 3 shows that 66.7% of the sealants were completely retained and 6.7% were completely lost after the 1-year follow-up. In considering the type of material, significantly more complete retentions were observed in the RBS group than in the GIC group (90.0% vs. 43.3%, $p = 0.01$). After the 1-year follow-up period, there were no dental caries lesions recorded in the second permanent molars sealed with RBSs or GIC.

After the 3-year follow-ups, the rates of partial retention (36.7%) and the complete loss of sealants (40.0%) were higher when compared with other outcome measurements, such as complete retention and filling. No complete retention of GIC sealants was found. Overall, 11.7% of the sealed occlusal surfaces were filled.

Table 3. Sealant retention characteristics according to the type of material over the whole follow-up period.

Follow-Up Period	Type of Material	Complete Retention, N (%)	Partial Retention, N (%)	Complete Loss, N (%)	Filling, N (%)	Total, N (%)	p-Value
1 year	RBS	27 (90.0) [a]	2 (6.7) [a]	1 (3.3)	0 (0.0)	30 (100.0)	
	GIC	13 (43.3) [a]	14 (46.7) [a]	3 (10.0)	0 (0.0)	30 (100.0)	0.01 [a]
	Total	40 (66.7)	16 (26.7)	4 (6.6)	0 (0.0)	60 (100.0)	
3 years	RBS	7 (23.3) [a]	11 (36.7)	9 (30.0)	3 (10.0)	30 (100.0)	
	GIC	0 (0.0) [a]	11 (36.7)	15 (50.0)	4 (13.3)	30 (100.0)	0.034 [a]
	Total	7 (11.7)	22 (36.6)	24 (40.0)	7 (11.7)	60 (100.0)	
10 years	RBS	2 (6.6)	8 (26.7)	11 (36.7)	9 (30.0)	30 (100.0)	
	GIC	0 (0.0)	3 (10.0)	16 (53.3)	11 (36.7)	30 (100.0)	0.145
	Total	2 (3.3)	11 (18.4)	27 (45.0)	20 (33.3)	60 (100.0)	

A chi-square test was conducted to compare the results of the sealant retention characteristics and both types of material during the follow-up periods. [a] significant difference between RBS and GIC. RBSs—resin-based sealants and GIC—glass ionomer cement.

The 10-year follow-ups showed that 6.7% of the RBSs were completely retained, while 36.7% of the RBSs and 53.3% of the GIC sealants were completely lost ($p = 0.145$) (Table 3). Subsequently, one-third of the sealed teeth (30.0% of the teeth sealed with RBSs and 36.7% of teeth applied with GIC) were already filled ($p = 0.145$) (Table 3).

Figure 3 shows the results of the Kaplan–Meier analysis, wherein it demonstrates the higher survival rate that was found in the RBS group when compared with the GIC group over the whole follow-up period ($p = 0.001$). Compared with RBSs, GIC sealants had a higher risk of failure; the hazard ratio (HR) was 1.426 (95% CI, 1.012–2.006, $p < 0.001$). Finally, the HR showed that the risk of caries development after sealant application with GIC was higher than with RBSs, although it did not differ statistically (1.250 (95% CI, 0.585–2.670 and $p = 0.565$)).

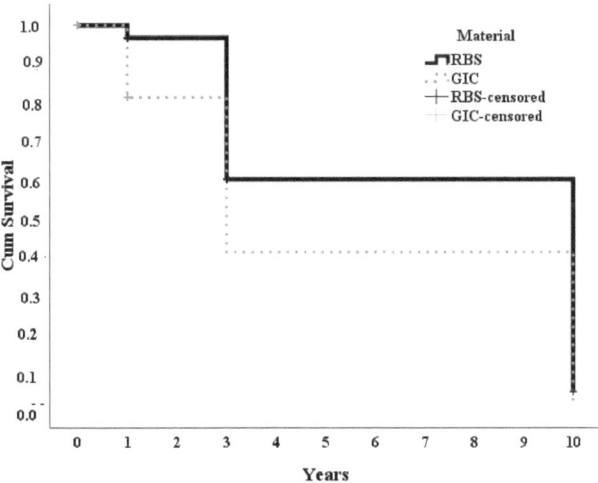

Figure 3. The cumulative survival curves for both types of sealants. "Failure" is defined as the loss of more than one-third of the sealant (via Log rank, $p = 0.001$).

Table 4 shows the rate of complete retention for both materials after the 1-year, 3-year, and 10-year follow-up periods with regard to the upper or lower teeth sealed. A higher complete retention rate of both materials was found on the maxillary permanent second molars during all three periods of follow-up ($p > 0.05$).

Table 4. Sealant retention characteristics as per the location of sealed teeth over the whole follow-up period.

Sealant Retention	Follow-Up					
	1 Year		3 Years		10 Years	
	RBS, N (%)	GIC, N (%)	RBS, N (%)	GIC, N (%)	RBS, N (%)	GIC, N (%)
Maxillary permanent second molars						
Complete retention	12 (92.3)	8 (47.1)	4 (30.8)	0 (0.0)	2 (15.4)	0 (0.0)
"Failure"	1 (7.7)	9 (52.9)	9 (69.2)	17 (100.0)	11 (84.6)	17 (100.0)
Total	13 (100.0)	17 (100.0)	13 (100.0)	17 (100.0)	13 (100.0)	17 (100.0)
Mandibular permanent second molars						
Complete retention	15 (88.2)	5 (38.5)	3 (17.6)	0 (0.0)	0 (0.0)	0 (0.0)
"Failure"	2 (11.8)	8 (61.5)	14 (82.4)	13 (100.0)	17 (100.0)	13 (100.0)
Total	17 (100.0)	13 (100.0)	17 (100.0)	13 (100.0)	17 (100.0)	13 (100.0)

A chi-square test was conducted to compare the results as per the tooth location and the sealant retention of both types of sealants during the follow-up periods ($p > 0.05$).

4. Discussion

The main finding of the study was the higher survival rate of resin-based sealants (RBSs) over glass ionomer cement (GIC) sealants when applied to second permanent molars over a long-term follow-up period. The clinical assessments of the sealant retention were performed after 1-year, 3-year, and 10-year periods. The participants' oral hygiene status was insignificantly improved and remained inadequate over the whole follow-up period. When considering the location, the complete sealant retention of both materials was insignificantly better on the maxillary permanent second molars over the whole period. In the present study, no caries lesion in the sealed second permanent molars was recorded during the 1-year follow-ups. After the 10-year follow-ups, the prevalence of the filled permanent second molars that had been previously applied with RBSs or GIC sealants did not differ significantly.

This study revealed that 90% of the RBSs were completely retained after a one-year follow-up period. Previous studies showed a high complete retention rate for RBSs, which varied from 62.5% to 96.7% after a 1-year follow-up period [3,42–44].

After three years, 23.3% of RBSs were completely retained in this study, while other studies reported a higher rate of complete retention of RBSs (which varied from 80.2% to 91.08% after the same period of follow-up [15,45]). The findings revealed that the complete or partial retention rate of GIC sealants was the same as it was found to be in another study performed by Hesse et al. [22].

When considering the 10-year follow-up period, half of the GIC sealants were completely lost, and 36.7% of the teeth applied with GIC sealants were already filled; these findings are in line with the results of another study carried out in Serbia [19]. Wendt et al. found that 65% of second permanent molars applied with resin-based sealants showed complete retention, and 5% of these teeth were found to be filled after 15-year follow-ups [27]. Long-term studies evaluating sealant retention are scarce [2].

This study revealed that the complete sealant retention of both materials was better on maxillary permanent second molars than on mandibular ones ($p > 0.05$). The same pattern of retention was observed in a study carried out in Romania [18]. Meanwhile, a study performed in Croatia showed the opposite results, i.e., better sealant retention on the mandibular molars ($p < 0.05$) [46].

The pit and fissure sealants' effectiveness was widely investigated in terms of retention, mechanical properties, different bonding, marginal microleakages, infiltration, and the emergence of caries, as detailed below [42,47–50]. This study employed the conventional acid etching protocol and cotton roll isolation technique during the sealant application procedure. Another study carried out in Lithuania compared the air abrasion and acid etching methods during RBS application and did not find significant differences in the sealant retention rate and caries development after 5-year follow-ups [42]. When considering bonding variations, the etch-and-rinse, multimode universal, and self-etch adhesives were used after acid etching, but the results did not confirm the effectiveness of the adhesive usage during RBS application after short-term follow-ups [47]. Meanwhile, another study revealed that an ethanol-based bonding agent being applied prior to resin-based sealant placement on first permanent molars significantly increased the retention at 12 months [48]. However, with respect to different isolation techniques, various studies have revealed opposite findings. Mattar et al. showed that the chosen type of isolation, such as the Isolite system, rubber dam, or cotton roll isolation, had no impact on the retention rate of pit and fissure sealants [49]; however, another study found that rubber dam isolation ensured better retention of sealants [50].

There are contradictory opinions regarding the clinical effectiveness of GIC sealants in caries prevention. GIC sealants have lower retention rates than RBSs [46,51,52], but the GIC material is more effective in occlusal caries prevention [51]. It has been found that GIC-based sealants applied according to the atraumatic restorative treatment (ART) protocol are effective at preventing dentine caries lesion development [52]. On the other hand, another study concluded that the application of GIC sealants on first permanent molars was not superior in reducing caries lesion development compared to non-applied molars [22]. However, the clinical relevance was focused not on sealant retention, but on the duration of potential caries prevention in previously sealed teeth [18]. Thus, GIC may be a proper material to seal recently erupted permanent molars for children in the high caries risk category when isolation of a tooth is challenging.

Long-term caries prevention strategies focus on non-operative caries treatment and sealant application, only for patients with high caries risk [29,30]. A high mean number of sealed teeth (4.29 [29] and 8.58 [30]) has indicated that oral health education, dietary counseling, personal tooth brushing, professional plaque removal, and fluoride varnish application may be insufficient measures in arresting caries progression for patients with low motivation [29,30]. These various implemented methods are effective in preventing caries development, although one intervention was not found to be more effective (superior) than another (varnish vs. sealant) [53,54].

The data from the National Oral Health Survey in Greece confirmed that sealant placement (low prevalence of sealants) is significantly associated with caries reduction (24%) in the 15-year-old group [55]. The sealant application for the first and second molars covered by the National Health Insurance Service contributed to decreasing dental caries in South Korea [56]. The financial resources of the national program for pit and fissure sealants in Lithuania were used inefficiently [33].

Numerous studies have proved that using merely professional dental measures, such as fluoride varnish or dental sealant applications, is not sufficient in avoiding dental caries development. Thus, oral hygiene instructions and dietary counseling play an essential role in dental caries prevention [57]. Regular supervised toothbrushing may be as efficient as the application of dental sealants in preventing dentin caries lesion development [58]. In considering long-term prognoses, the most favorable results were achieved when dental sealants were integrated as a component in caries prevention programs [59].

Strength and Limitation

The main strengths of this study need to be considered. The long-term follow-up for the evaluation of sealant retention and caries development may be considered as the main advantage of this study. However, a relatively small sample size was one of the limitations of this study. The split mouth design was not used, although bitewing radiographs were taken prior to the application of sealants. Furthermore, other methods, such as fiber optic transillumination and laser fluorescence, were not employed to detect occlusal caries.

5. Conclusions

Although the survival rate of RBSs was higher than that of GIC sealants, their effectiveness in preventing fissure caries in permanent second molars did not differ significantly over a 10-year follow-up period. Glass ionomer sealants could be a good alternative as an initial temporary sealant material due to better moisture tolerance than resin-based sealants when optimal saliva control during sealant application is not feasible.

Author Contributions: Conceptualization and methodology, K.S.-M. and J.N.; investigation, K.S.-M.; data writing—original draft preparation, S.P.; writing—review and editing, S.P., K.S.-M., and J.N.; visualization, S.P., K.S.-M., and J.N.; supervision, J.N. All authors have read and agreed to the published version of the manuscript.

Funding: This research received no external funding.

Institutional Review Board Statement: This study was conducted in accordance with the guidelines detailed in the Declaration of Helsinki. The Kaunas Regional Biomedical Research Ethics Committee approved the study protocol (no. 100/2003-12-03), and the parents of the participants provided their written informed consent to participate in the study.

Informed Consent Statement: Informed consent was obtained from all parents of subjects involved in the study.

Data Availability Statement: The data presented in this study are available from the corresponding authors.

Conflicts of Interest: The authors declare no conflicts of interest.

References

1. Carvalho, J.C.; Dige, I.; Machiulskiene, V.; Qvist, V.; Bakhshandeh, A.; Fatturi-Parolo, C.; Maltz, M. Occlusal Caries: Biological Approach for Its Diagnosis and Management. *Caries Res.* **2016**, *50*, 527–542. [CrossRef] [PubMed]
2. Ng, T.C.; Chu, C.H.; Yu, O.Y. A concise review of dental sealants in caries management. *Front. Oral Health* **2023**, *4*, 1180405. [CrossRef] [PubMed]
3. Berescescu, L.; Păcurar, M.; Bica, C.I.; Vlasa, A.; Stoica, O.E.; Dako, T.; Petcu, B.; Esian, D. The Assessment of Sealants' Effectiveness in Arresting Non-Cavitated Caries Lesion-A 24-Month Follow-Up. *Healthcare* **2022**, *10*, 1651. [CrossRef] [PubMed]
4. Centers for Disease Control and Prevention Division of Oral Health. Dental Sealants. 2013. Available online: https://www.cdc.gov/oralhealth/dental_sealant_program/sealants-FAQ.htm (accessed on 31 March 2015).
5. Handelman, S.L.; Buonocore, M.G.; Heseck, D.J. A preliminary report on the effect of fissure sealant on bacteria in dental caries. *J. Prosthet. Dent.* **1972**, *27*, 390–392. [CrossRef] [PubMed]
6. Simonsen, R.J. Pit and fissure sealants. In *Clinical Applications of the Acid Etch Technique*; Quintessence Publishing Co. Inc.: Chicago, IL, USA, 1978; pp. 19–42.
7. Ahovuo-Saloranta, A.; Forss, H.; Walsh, T.; Nordblad, A.; Mäkelä, M.; Worthington, H.V. Pit and fissure sealants for preventing dental decay in permanent teeth. *Cochrane Database Syst. Rev.* **2017**, *7*, CD001830. [CrossRef] [PubMed]
8. Carvalho, J.C.; Figueredo, C.S.; Mestrinho, H.D. Clinical report on plaque formation, distribution and maturation within the primary, mixed and permanent dentitions. *Eur. J. Paediatr. Dent.* **2009**, *10*, 193–199. [PubMed]
9. Ahovuo-Saloranta, A.; Forss, H.; Hiiri, A.; Nordblad, A.; Mäkelä, M. Pit and fissure sealants versus fluoride varnishes for preventing dental decay in the permanent teeth of children and adolescents. *Cochrane Database Syst. Rev.* **2016**, *2016*, CD003067. [CrossRef] [PubMed]
10. Alsabek, L.; Al-Nerabieah, Z.; Bshara, N.; Comisi, J.C. Retention and remineralization effect of moisture tolerant resin-based sealant and glass ionomer sealant on non-cavitated pit and fissure caries: Randomized controlled clinical trial. *J. Dent.* **2019**, *86*, 69–74. [CrossRef]
11. Cvikl, B.; Moritz, A.; Bekes, K. Pit and Fissure Sealants-A Comprehensive Review. *Dent. J.* **2018**, *6*, 18. [CrossRef]

12. Buonocore, M.G. A simple method of increasing the adhesion of acrylic filling materials to enamel surfaces. *J. Dent. Res.* **1955**, *34*, 849–853. [CrossRef]
13. McLean, J.W.; Wilson, A.D. Fissure sealing and filling with an adhesive glass-ionomer cement. *Br. Dent. J.* **1974**, *136*, 269–276. [CrossRef] [PubMed]
14. Uzel, I.; Gurlek, C.; Kuter, B.; Ertugrul, F.; Eden, E. Caries-Preventive Effect and Retention of Glass-Ionomer and Resin-Based Sealants: A Randomized Clinical Comparative Evaluation. *Biomed. Res. Int.* **2022**, *2022*, 7205692. [CrossRef] [PubMed]
15. Ozan, G.; Sancakli, H.S.; Erdemir, U.; Yaman, B.C.; Yildiz, S.O.; Yildiz, E. Comparative evaluation of a fissure sealant and a flowable composite: A 36-month split-mouth, randomized clinical study. *J. Dent.* **2022**, *123*, 104205. [CrossRef] [PubMed]
16. Kühnisch, J.; Mansmann, U.; Heinrich-Weltzien, R.; Hickel, R. Longevity of materials for pit and fissure sealing--results from a meta-analysis. *Dent. Mater.* **2012**, *28*, 298–303. [CrossRef] [PubMed]
17. Lam, P.P.; Sardana, D.; Lo, E.C.; Yiu, C.K. Fissure sealant in a nutshell. evidence-based meta-evaluation of sealants' effectiveness in caries prevention and arrest. *J. Evid. Based Dent. Pract.* **2021**, *21*, 101587. [CrossRef] [PubMed]
18. Muntean, A.; Sarosi, C.; Sava, S.; Moldovan, M.; Condurache, A.I.; Delean, A.G. Dental Sealant Composition-Retention Assessment in Young Permanent Molars. *Materials* **2021**, *14*, 1646. [CrossRef]
19. Markovic, D.; Peric, T.; Petrovic, B. Glass-ionomer fissure sealants: Clinical observations up to 13 years. *J. Dent.* **2018**, *79*, 85–89. [CrossRef]
20. Colombo, S.; Beretta, M. Dental Sealants Part 3: Which material? Efficiency and effectiveness. *Eur. J. Paediatr. Dent.* **2018**, *19*, 247–249. [CrossRef]
21. Sly, G.E.; Missana, L.R.; Nieva, N.; Kaplan, A.E. Ex vivo microleakage comparison between glass ionomers used as pit and fissure sealants. *Acta Odontol. Latinoam.* **2015**, *28*, 132–137.
22. Hesse, D.; Guglielmi, C.A.B.; Raggio, D.P.; Bönecker, M.J.S.; Mendes, F.M.; Bonifácio, C.C. Atraumatic Restorative Treatment-Sealed versus Nonsealed First Permanent Molars: A 3-Year Split-Mouth Clinical Trial. *Caries Res.* **2021**, *55*, 12–20. [CrossRef]
23. Bhushan, U.; Goswami, M. Evaluation of retention of pit and fissure sealants placed with and without air abrasion pretreatment in 6–8 year old children—An in vivo study. *J. Clin. Exp. Dent.* **2017**, *9*, e211–e217. [CrossRef] [PubMed]
24. Botton, G.; Morgental, C.S.; Scherer, M.M.; Lenzi, T.L.; Montagner, A.F.; Rocha, R.O. Are self-etch adhesive systems effective in the retention of occlusal sealants? A systematic review and meta-analysis. *Int. J. Paediatr. Dent.* **2016**, *26*, 402–411. [CrossRef] [PubMed]
25. Azarpazhooh, A.; Main, P.A. Pit and fissure sealants in the prevention of dental caries in children and adolescents: A systematic review. *J. Can. Dent. Assoc.* **2008**, *74*, 171–177. [PubMed]
26. Bakhtiar, M.; Azadi, N.; Golkari, A. One-Year Evaluation of a Free Fissure Sealant Program. *J. Dent. Biomater.* **2016**, *3*, 306–314.
27. Wendt, L.K.; Koch, G.; Birkhed, D. On the retention and effectiveness of fissure sealant in permanent molars after 15–20 years: A cohort study. *Community Dent. Oral Epidemiol.* **2001**, *29*, 302–307. [CrossRef] [PubMed]
28. Soto-Rojas, A.E.; Escoffié-Ramírez, M.; Pérez-Ferrera, G.; Guido, J.A.; Mantilla-Rodriguez, A.A.; Martinez-Mier, E.A. Retention of dental sealants placed on sound teeth and incipient caries lesions as part of a service-learning programme in rural areas in Mexico. *Int. J. Paediatr. Dent.* **2012**, *22*, 451–458. [CrossRef]
29. Ekstrand, K.R.; Christiansen, M.E. Outcomes of a non-operative caries treatment programme for children and adolescents. *Caries Res.* **2005**, *39*, 455–467. [CrossRef]
30. Ekstrand, K.R.; Abreu-Placeres, N. The impact of a national caries strategy in Greenland 10 years after implementation. A failure or a success? *Int. J. Circumpolar Health* **2020**, *79*, 1804260. [CrossRef]
31. Children's Health Monitoring System. Available online: https://vssis.hi.lt/Naujienos/Naujiena?NewsId=1415 (accessed on 9 January 2024).
32. Mačiulskienė, V.; Razmienė, J.; Andruškevičienė, V.; Bendoraitienė, E. Estimation of Caries Treatment Needs in First Permanent Molars of Lithuanian 5–6-Year-Old Children, Based on Caries Lesion Activity Assessment. *Medicina* **2020**, *56*, 105. [CrossRef]
33. Saldūnaite, K.; Pūrienė, A.; Milčiuvienė, S.; Brukiene, V.; Kutkauskiene, J. Analysis of dental caries prevention program in 7–12-year-old Lithuanian schoolchildren. *Medicina* **2009**, *45*, 887–895. (In Lithuanian) [CrossRef]
34. Milciuviene, S.; Bendoraitiene, E.; Andruskeviciene, V.; Narbutaite, J.; Sakalauskiene, J.; Vasiliauskiene, I.; Slabsinskiene, E. Dental caries prevalence among 12–15-year-olds in Lithuania between 1983 and 2005. *Medicina* **2009**, *45*, 68–76. [CrossRef] [PubMed]
35. Machiulskiene, V.; Nyvad, B.; Baelum, V. Prevalence and severity of dental caries in 12-year-old children in Kaunas, Lithuania 1995. *Caries Res.* **1998**, *32*, 175–180. [CrossRef] [PubMed]
36. The Order of the Minister of Health of the Republic of Lithuania. Description of the Budgetary Procedure for Covering Children's Molars with Silant Materials and Reimbursement of Expenses from the Compulsory Health Insurance Fund. 2005. Available online: https://e-seimas.lrs.lt/portal/legalAct/lt/TAD/TAIS.262507/PHbgIHxRFd (accessed on 7 March 2023).
37. World Health Organization. *Oral Health Surveys: Basic Methods*, 4th ed.; World Health Organization: Geneva, Switzerland, 1997.
38. Wilkins, E.M. *Clinical Practice of the Dental Hygienist*, 7th ed.; LesFebiger: Washington, DC, USA, 1994; pp. 289–290.
39. World Health Organization. *Oral Health Surveys: Basic Methods*, 5th ed.; World Health Organization: Geneva, Switzerland, 2013.
40. Kilpatrick, N.M.; Murray, J.J.; McCabe, J.F. A clinical comparison of a light cured glass ionomer sealant restoration with a composite sealant restoration. *J. Dent.* **1996**, *24*, 399–405. [CrossRef] [PubMed]
41. Kashbour, W.; Gupta, P.; Worthington, H.V.; Boyers, D. Pit and fissure sealants versus fluoride varnishes for preventing dental decay in the permanent teeth of children and adolescents. *Cochrane Database Syst. Rev.* **2020**, *11*, CD003067. [CrossRef] [PubMed]

42. Bendinskaite, R.; Peciuliene, V.; Brukiene, V. A five years clinical evaluation of sealed occlusal surfaces of molars. *Stomatologija* **2010**, *12*, 87–92. [PubMed]
43. Hassan, A.M.; Mohammed, S.G. Effectiveness of Seven Types of Sealants: Retention after One Year. *Int. J. Clin. Pediatr. Dent.* **2019**, *12*, 96–100. [CrossRef] [PubMed]
44. Behroozian, A.; Aghazadeh, Z.; Sadrabad, Z.K.; Aghazadeh, M.; Alizadeh, V.; Esmaili, Z.; Pirzadeh Ashraf, M. Evaluation of the success rate of pit and fissure sealants on first molars: 12 months follow-up study. *Int. J. Dent. Hyg.* **2022**, *20*, 465–470. [CrossRef]
45. Baseggio, W.; Naufel, F.S.; Davidoff, D.C.; Nahsan, F.P.; Flury, S.; Rodrigues, J.A. Caries-preventive efficacy and retention of a resin-modified glass ionomer cement and a resin-based fissure sealant: A 3-year split-mouth randomised clinical trial. *Oral Health Prev. Dent.* **2010**, *8*, 261–268.
46. Reić, T.; Galić, T.; Negovetić, V.D. Retention and caries-preventive effect of four different sealant materials: A 2-year prospective split-mouth study. *Int. J. Paediatr. Dent.* **2022**, *32*, 449–457. [CrossRef]
47. Khare, M.; Suprabha, B.S.; Shenoy, R.; Rao, A. Evaluation of pit-and-fissure sealants placed with four different bonding protocols: A randomized clinical trial. *Int. J. Paediatr. Dent.* **2017**, *27*, 444–453. [CrossRef]
48. McCafferty, J.; O'Connell, A.C. A randomised clinical trial on the use of intermediate bonding on the retention of fissure sealants in children. *Int. J. Paediatr. Dent.* **2016**, *26*, 110–115. [CrossRef] [PubMed]
49. Mattar, R.E.; Sulimany, A.M.; Binsaleh, S.S.; Hamdan, H.M.; Al-Majed, I.M. Evaluation of fissure sealant retention rates using Isolite in comparison with rubber dam and cotton roll isolation techniques: A randomized clinical trial. *Int. J. Paediatr. Dent.* **2023**, *33*, 12–19. [CrossRef] [PubMed]
50. Cortez, T.V.; Godoy, E.P.; Paschoini, V.L.; Corona, S.A.M.; Borsatto, M.C.; Souza-Gabriel, A.E. Clinical performance of sealants under different humidity control conditions: A split-mouth 1-year randomized trial. *Eur. Arch. Paediatr. Dent.* **2023**, *24*, 769–777. [CrossRef] [PubMed]
51. Ulusu, T.; Odabaş, M.E.; Tüzüner, T.; Baygin, O.; Sillelioğlu, H.; Deveci, C.; Gökdoğan, F.G.; Altuntaş, A. The success rates of a glass ionomer cement and a resin-based fissure sealant placed by fifth-year undergraduate dental students. *Eur. Arch. Paediatr. Dent.* **2012**, *13*, 94–97. [CrossRef] [PubMed]
52. Liu, B.Y.; Xiao, Y.; Chu, C.H.; Lo, E.C. Glass ionomer ART sealant and fluoride-releasing resin sealant in fissure caries prevention—Results from a randomized clinical trial. *BMC Oral Health* **2014**, *14*, 54. [CrossRef] [PubMed]
53. Chestnutt, I.G.; Playle, R.; Hutchings, S.; Morgan-Trimmer, S.; Fitzsimmons, D.; Aawar, N.; Angel, L.; Derrick, S.; Drew, C.; Hoddell, C.; et al. Fissure Seal or Fluoride Varnish? A Randomized Trial of Relative Effectiveness. *J. Dent. Res.* **2017**, *96*, 754–761. [CrossRef] [PubMed]
54. Uchil, S.R.; Suprabha, B.S.; Shenoy, R.; Rao, A. Clinical effectiveness of resin-modified glass ionomer-based fluoride varnish for preventing occlusal caries lesions in partially erupted permanent molars: A randomised active-controlled trial. *Int. J. Paediatr. Dent.* **2022**, *32*, 314–323. [CrossRef] [PubMed]
55. Oulis, C.J.; Berdouses, E.D.; Mamai-Homata, E.; Polychronopoulou, A. Prevalence of sealants in relation to dental caries on the permanent molars of 12 and 15-year-old Greek adolescents. A national pathfinder survey. *BMC Public Health* **2011**, *11*, 100. [CrossRef]
56. Choi, J.S.; Ma, D.S. Changes in oral health indicators due to implementation of the National Health Insurance Services coverage for first molar dental sealant for children and adolescents in South Korea. *BMC Oral Health* **2020**, *20*, 214. [CrossRef]
57. Paglia, L.; Ferrazzano, G.; Beretta, M. The Role of Pit and Fissure Sealants in the Prevention of Dental Caries. In *Pit and Fissure Sealants*; Bekes, K., Ed.; Springer: Cham, Switzerland, 2018.
58. Hilgert, L.A.; Leal, S.C.; Mulder, J.; Creugers, N.H.; Frencken, J.E. Caries-preventive Effect of Supervised Toothbrushing and Sealants. *J. Dent. Res.* **2015**, *94*, 1218–1224. [CrossRef]
59. Splieth, C.H.; Ekstrand, K.R.; Alkilzy, M.; Clarkson, J.; Meyer-Lueckel, H.; Martignon, S.; Paris, S.; Pitts, N.B.; Ricketts, D.N.; van Loveren, C. Sealants in dentistry: Outcomes of the ORCA Saturday Afternoon Symposium 2007. *Caries Res.* **2010**, *44*, 3–13. [CrossRef] [PubMed]

Disclaimer/Publisher's Note: The statements, opinions and data contained in all publications are solely those of the individual author(s) and contributor(s) and not of MDPI and/or the editor(s). MDPI and/or the editor(s) disclaim responsibility for any injury to people or property resulting from any ideas, methods, instructions or products referred to in the content.

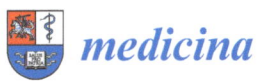

Article

Comparative Meta-Analysis of Minimally Invasive and Conventional Approaches for Caries Removal in Permanent Dentition

Diego González-Gil [1], Javier Flores-Fraile [1,*], Vicente Vera-Rodríguez [2], Andrea Martín-Vacas [3] and Joaquín López-Marcos [1]

1. Dental Clinic Faculty of Medicine, Surgery Department, University of Salamanca, 37007 Salamanca, Spain; diegoggil@usal.es (D.G.-G.); jflmarcos@usal.es (J.L.-M.)
2. TUFTS Dental School, Boston, MA 02155, USA; vicente.vera_rodriguez@tufts.edu
3. Faculty of Dentistry, Alfonso X El Sabio University, 28691 Madrid, Spain; amartvac@uax.es
* Correspondence: j.flores@usal.es

Citation: González-Gil, D.; Flores-Fraile, J.; Vera-Rodríguez, V.; Martín-Vacas, A.; López-Marcos, J. Comparative Meta-Analysis of Minimally Invasive and Conventional Approaches for Caries Removal in Permanent Dentition. *Medicina* **2024**, *60*, 402. https://doi.org/10.3390/medicina60030402

Academic Editor: Bruno Chrcanovic

Received: 4 January 2024
Revised: 13 February 2024
Accepted: 22 February 2024
Published: 27 February 2024

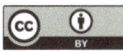

Copyright: © 2024 by the authors. Licensee MDPI, Basel, Switzerland. This article is an open access article distributed under the terms and conditions of the Creative Commons Attribution (CC BY) license (https://creativecommons.org/licenses/by/4.0/).

Abstract: *Background and Objectives:* Addressing deep carious lesions poses significant challenges in daily dental practice due to the inherent complexity of their treatment. Traditionally, complete removal of carious tissues has been the norm, potentially leading to pulp tissue exposure and subsequent pulpitis. In contemporary dentistry, there is a growing preference for minimally invasive techniques, such as selective removal, offering a more conservative approach with enhanced predictability and success rates. *Materials and Methods:* Our study commenced with a comprehensive systematic review. After that, we performed a meta-analysis focused exclusively on randomized controlled trials involving permanent dentition. Our investigation incorporated seven selected articles, which scrutinized success rates and the incidence of pulp exposure in minimally invasive techniques (MIT) versus conventional techniques (CT). Statistical analysis employed U Mann–Whitney and Wilcoxon tests to interpret the results. *Results:* Although the difference did not reach statistical significance, MIT demonstrated marginally superior success rates compared to CT. Furthermore, MIT exhibited a lower percentage of pulp exposure when contrasted with CT. However, due to the limited sample size, statistical significance for this difference could not be established. *Conclusions:* Minimally invasive techniques for caries removal emerge as a conservative and promising approach to safeguard pulp tissues in comparison to conventional techniques. The need for additional randomized controlled trials is emphasized to unequivocally establish the superior success rates of these procedures over their conventional counterparts.

Keywords: selective caries removal; incomplete caries removal

1. Introduction

Dental caries is a biofilm-mediated, diet modulated, multifactorial, dynamic disease resulting in mineral loss of dental hard tissues [1]. Nowadays, this disease is widespread throughout the world, affecting billions of teeth [2–4]. When caries produces very deep lesions in dentin, dental pulp can be damaged, compromising its vitality. Over the years, dentists have faced the challenge of knowing how much dentin to remove or preserve in order to perform a proper treatment [5–8]. During the 19th century, G.V. Black suggested that carious tissue should be removed until sound physiological dentin was reached, although this procedure may lead to pulp exposure. Almost a century later, Fusuyama improved caries removal techniques by recognizing two different types of dentine: inner demineralized zone or affected dentin and outer contaminated or infected dentine [9,10]. The inner zone presents a firm consistence, as there is a little resistance while removing it. As this zone is susceptible to remineralization, it should be respected and maintained.

The outer zone presents soft dentin as it is highly contaminated, and should be completely removed during our restorative procedures [11].

Traditionally, complete caries removal procedures such as stepwise technique have been used to remove deep caries in a non-selective way. Stepwise technique consists of the elimination of both firm and soft dentin in deep caries removal. This procedure may cause pulp exposure and excessive removal of tooth structure, and it is performed in two different visits by placing a temporary restoration between appointments. This conventional method presents some disadvantages; for instance, a high risk of irreversible pulp damage, which results in higher costs to the patient, or an increase in office visits [6,12,13].

Nowadays, minimally invasive dentistry should be a guide mark to restore dental caries and there are new procedures that offer advantages over conventional methods. Although selective procedures are well documented in the literature, with respect to deciduous teeth, there are few investigations about these techniques in permanent dentition [14]. Since both dentitions present differences, such as size of teeth or regenerative potential, they should be studied separately. Selective caries removal to soft or firm dentine is less invasive than stepwise technique, and it offers great results. This method is also known as incomplete caries removal technique, and it pretends to respect pulp tissues by not eliminating soft dentin near the pulp chamber [15–22]. While removing decay, procedures such as caries dyes or laser fluorescence can be used to perform a proper selective technique. Caries detector dyes stain outer and inner zones differently, in order to distinguish them. However, this procedure may lead to excessive tissue removal, as it is not accurate in assessing the amount of contamination present in each zone [23,24]. Another product that is used during selective caries removal is Cariosolv, which is a gel that removes contaminated dentin, respecting demineralized tissues. This procedure, when combined with a microscope, can be a great alternative to restore deep caries [25–28]. On the other hand, the DIAGNOdent pen uses fluorescence technology for the detection of bacterial porphyrins and it provides useful information about dentin contamination [29]. Another effective procedure using laser fluorescence during selective caries removal is the FACE device, which consists of an orange-red laser that allows recognition of highly contaminated areas [30,31]. Tactile evaluation of tissue hardness should be taken into account along with laser fluorescence and caries detector dyes as effective methods to achieve a proper selective treatment [10,32,33].

While performing selective caries removal, it is important to follow a great bonding protocol to obtain successful long-term restorations [12,34,35]. Only sound dentin allows an adequate bond strength, as inner and outer dentin present high percentages of bond strength loss from 25% to 66%, respectively. This important decrease in values is due to the great demineralization in these carious zones [36–38]. A key point to accomplish a suitable bond strength is to create a peripheral seal zone 1 to 3 mm wide, free from soft dentin. Caries detector dyes and fluorescence techniques will help us to confirm the absence of contaminated dentin outside our peripheral seal zone. Highly infected dentin inside our seal area should be eliminated without exposing pulp chamber. Regarding the bonding system, it is recommended to use a three-step total etch or a mild two-step self-etching in order to obtain a great bond strength during selective caries removal [9,10]. With this investigation, we pretend to compare success rates in minimally invasive techniques and conventional procedures in order to know which one offers better results, as well as studying pulp exposure in both techniques to evaluate its influence in success rates.

2. Materials and Methods

2.1. Study Desing

We performed a systematic review of randomized controlled trials that studied selective caries removal techniques and showed results of pulp exposure and success rates in permanent dentition, including articles from the period from January 2008 to December 2022, covering only articles published in English. After that, we conducted a meta-analysis with those articles that met our study requirements. We carried out a study selection according to the Preferred Reporting Items for Systematic Review and Meta-Analyses (PRISMA) guidelines for reporting systematic reviews. This investigation is property registered with in Prospero database with this code: CRD42023390509 Prospero Register Code.

The search strategy was conducted using the population, intervention, comparison, and outcome (PICO) framework based on the following question: "is the success rate of selective caries removal techniques better than conventional ones?"

2.2. Inclusion Criteria

We have only included randomized controlled trials that compared selective and non-selective techniques of caries removal in permanent teeth, as well as articles written in English and with the full text available.

2.3. Exclusion Criteria

After conducting the systematic review and reviewing titles and abstracts of selective procedures, we observed that the majority of investigations were focused on primary dentition. Consequently, all articles that examined techniques in primary dentition were excluded, as well as unfinished trials. This process is illustrated in the flowchart (Figure 1).

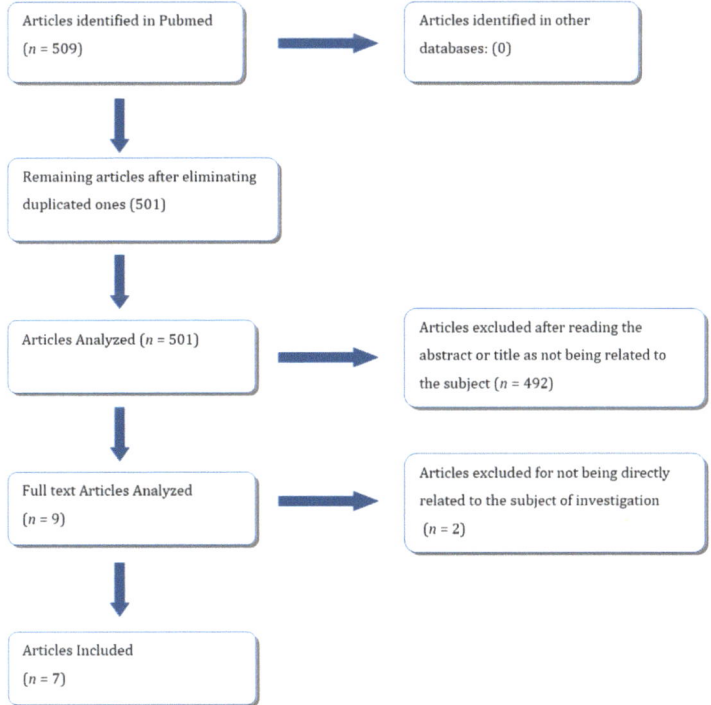

Figure 1. Flowchart showing systematic review.

2.4. Variables

After obtaining values of each kind of technique, we established a comparison between them in order to know which one offers better results. All data was analyzed statistically.

Quality Assessment of the Included Studies

The risk of bias of each included study was estimated using the Cochrane risk bias assessment tool, as it is represented in Figure 2. Most of these studies present a low risk of bias, especially those that are more recent. Studies such as Jardim, Labib, or Maltz focus on a type of procedure that must be performed in two appointments, making it impossible to blind patients. Casagrande's study is retrospective, which makes some of the risk of bias domains challenging to measure. However, random sequence generation, allocation concealment, blinding, and reporting are well performed in these investigations.

Author and year	Goezetici 2022	Jardim 2020	Labib 2019	Ali 2018	Kohkar 2018	Maltz 2018	Casagrande 2017
Random sequence generation	✓	✓	✓	✓	✓	✓	?
Allocation concealment	✓	✓	✓	✓	✓	✓	✓
Blinding of participants	✓	?	?	✓	?	✗	✗
Blinding of outcome assessment	✓	✓	✓	?	?	?	✓
Incomplete outcome data	✓	✓	?	✓	✓	✓	✗
Selective reporting	✓	✓	✓	✓	?	✓	✓

Figure 2. Quality assessments of included studies: ✓ indicates low risk of bias; ? represents an unclear risk of bias; ✗ represents a high risk of bias [39–45].

2.5. Statistical Analysis

With respect to statistical analysis, we included normality test of quantitative variables in order to apply parametric or no-parametric tests. If the data number is greater than 50, we considered using a Kolmogorov–Smirnov test; or a Shapiro–Wilk test, in cases where this value is less than 50. We performed a comparison of mean values of distribution in quantitative variable of each group, that is determined by qualitative variable. When this variable presents two categories, Student's t test should be used, but in this case, we applied the Mann–Whitney U non-parametric test, as there is a small sample. We used paired sample test to prove if it is possible to accept, with 95% confidence, that there is a statistical difference between variables. In this investigation, there is a small sample, so we used the Wilcoxon non-parametric test. All statistical test were applied with a confidence level of 95% by using SPSS version 26.0 software.

2.6. Resources

Bibliographical Resources

Medical Database Pubmed-Medline was consulted, and social media ResearchGate was used as a complement in order to obtain some full-text articles.

The key words used were "selective caries removal" and "incomplete caries removal". A cross-search was also performed using these terms: "selective caries removal and permanent".

3. Results

After performing a complete review in the literature, only seven articles were included in this metanalysis, as there are very few randomized trial controls that study the comparison of different caries removal procedures in permanent dentition. Besides this, there is a lack of homogeneity in conventional and minimally invasive methods as we had to mix similar procedures with variations in their protocols. In this manner, we categorized these techniques into two types: minimally invasive techniques (MIT), which encompass selective caries removal to soft dentin, self-limiting techniques, and incomplete caries removal. On the other hand, within conventional techniques (CT), we included selective caries removal to firm dentin, step-wise techniques, and complete caries removal.

The results of the metanalysis are represented in Table 1. This table shows the sample and the follow-up of every investigation, as well as a brief description of each technique. Also, the percentages of success rate and pulp exposure are represented in the articles that measured these values. Success rates comparisons of minimally invasive techniques and conventional techniques are shown in Figure 3. Figures 4 and 5 show pulp exposure rates in MIT and in CT. Not all investigations studied pulp exposure, so there is a lack of figures in those columns. The Mann–Whitney Test indicated no significant difference between both techniques, with a result of 0.2 (*p*-value > 0.05). The Wilcoxon Test yielded a value of 0.0, which is in close proximity to our significance threshold (*p*-value = 0.068).

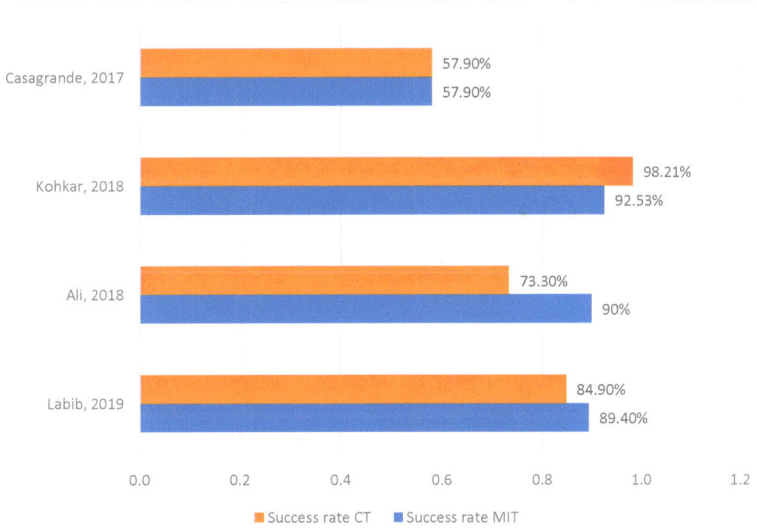

Figure 3. Success rate comparison [41–43,45].

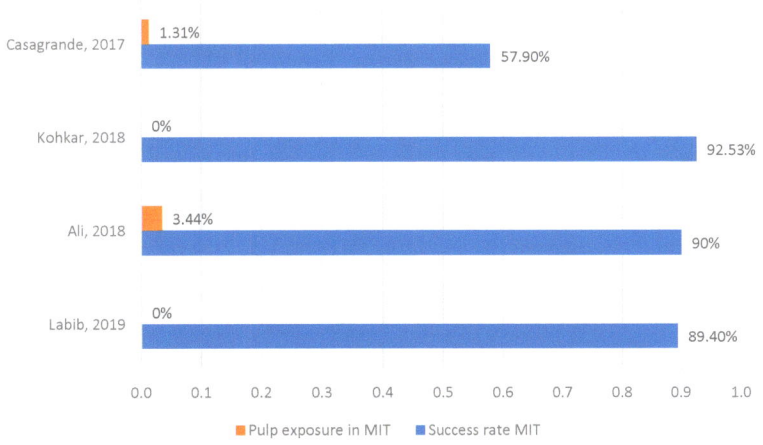

Figure 4. Pulp exposure and success rate in MIT [41–43,45].

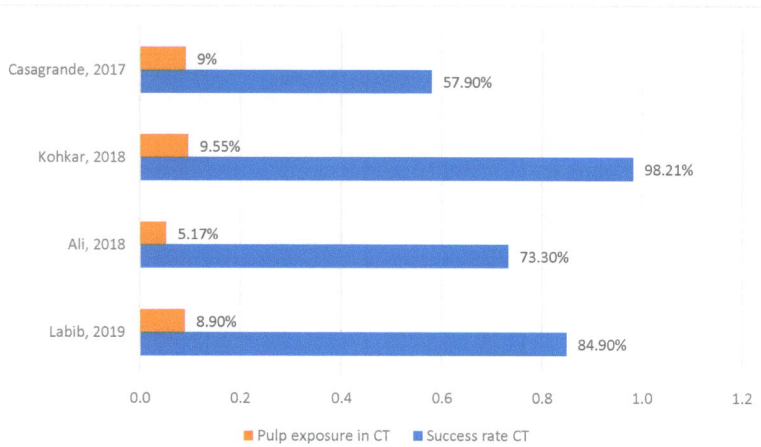

Figure 5. Pulp exposure and success rate in CT [41–43,45].

Table 1. Articles meta-analyzed.

Study and Year	Sample	Follow-Up	Minimally Invasive Technique	vs.	Conventional Technique	Success Rate MIT	Success Rate CT	Pulp Exposure in MIT	Pulp Exposure in CT
Goezetici, 2022 [39]	113 restorations	2 years	Selective removal to soft dentin: an amount of carious tissue was left over the pulp		Selective removal to firm dentin: carious tissue was completely removed	96.7%	83.2%	-	-
Jardim, 2020 [40]	172 restorations	5 years	Selective removal to soft dentin: only disorganized dentin was removed		Stepwise excavation: two-step complete caries removal	79%	76%	-	-
Labib, 2019 [41]	106 restorations	1 year	Selective caries removal in one step		Stepwise excavation: two-step complete caries removal	89.4%	84.9%	0%	8.9%
Ali, 2018 [42]	85 restorations	1 year	Self-limiting technique: use of microscope combined with chemo mechanical excavation		Conventional technique: subjective removal to leathery dentin	90%	73.3%	3.4%	5.2%
Kohkar, 2018 [43]	123 restorations	1, 5 years	Partial caries removal: soft dentin was left over the pulp		Complete caries removal	92.5%	98%	0%	9.5%
Maltz, 2018 [44]	229 restorations	5 years	Partial Caries removal: selective caries removal in one session		Stepwise excavation: two-step complete caries removal	80%	56%	-	-
Casagrande, 2017 [45]	477 restorations	3 years	Selective caries removal		Complete caries removal in one session	57.9%	57.9%	1.2%	9%

4. Discussion

While performing this meta-analysis, we realized how scarce the literature is regarding the comparison between selective and non-selective removal procedures in permanent dentition. Although there are several randomized control trials on primary teeth [46–49], it is very difficult to find these types of investigations on permanent teeth. Furthermore, some of these studies on permanent teeth are still unfinished [50,51]. Another complication during this investigation was the lack of homogeneity of all techniques, which forced us to include similar procedures that presented variations in their protocols in the same study group [39–45]. We believe that further research should be conducted to investigate various techniques in order to establish a gold standard method that unifies proven successful protocols for the selective treatment of caries. A comprehensive exploration of these methods will contribute to the development of standardized techniques that guide our treatments in a minimally invasive direction, reducing trauma and costs for the patient.

Nowadays, minimally invasive dentistry, as well as biomimetic dentistry, has gained a lot of importance in our dental offices. However, when it comes to the treatment of caries, the majority of professionals still prefer to use conventional techniques, and there is limited documentation in the literature. According to this new treatment philosophy, we aim to be as conservative as possible with dental tissues. Specifically, when referring to caries removal, we should try to preserve the dental pulp and maintain the vitality of the affected tooth [2,3].

With this investigation, we aim to compare if minimally invasive caries removal techniques present better results than conventional ones and if pulp exposure that may occur while performing these procedures may influence their success. All the articles we analyzed present a comparison between a less invasive technique and another more invasive one, so we divided the procedure into two kinds: minimally invasive techniques and conventional techniques. In minimally invasive techniques (MIT), we included the following procedures: selective caries removal to soft dentin in one step [39–41,45], self-limiting technique [42] and partial caries removal [43,44]. All of these procedures are associated with conservative dentistry and demonstrate a high level of respect for pulp tissue. The self-limiting technique consists of an experimental protocol that combines the use of a clinical microscope with the chemomechanical removal of deep carious tissue using Cariosolv gel [42]. In conventional techniques (CT) we considered the following: selective caries removal to firm dentin [38], step-wise excavation [40,41,44] and complete caries removal [42,43,45]. Both selective caries removal to firm dentin and complete caries removal are too invasive as they do not respect affected dentin at the pulp wall. In these conventional procedures, all affected and infected dentin is removed from the cavity, even though pulp exposure may occur.

The step-wise procedure is based on the elimination of decayed tissue in two appointments. During the initial visit, carious dentin is excavated from the surrounding walls while maintaining affected dentin at the pulpal wall. Subsequently, a temporary seal is applied for 6 or 9 months, aiming to isolate microorganisms and control caries progression. In a follow-up visit, the cavity is reopened to complete the excavation, and the final restoration is placed [43]. Although this technique is more respectful to pulp tissues than complete removal procedures, it is not considered a minimally invasive procedure due to the duration of the temporary restoration and the increased number of dental appointments. As evidenced in the literature reviewed for this investigation, minimally invasive techniques yield excellent results within a shorter procedural time, sparing the patient from the need for two complex appointments. On the other hand, complete caries removal is a traditional technique that is less conservative and may cause harm to the pulp in many cases. By opting for selective caries removal, we can preserve pulp vitality, thereby avoiding the need for endodontic treatment, which is a significant benefit for the patient.

Initially, we compared the success rates of minimally invasive techniques (MIT) with those of conventional techniques (CT). Mean values in MIT (83.6%) are higher than CT ones [75.4%], indicating that selective techniques seem to be slightly more effective than conventional ones. By analyzing these results, it becomes evident that minimally invasive techniques are a superior alternative to conventional techniques when treating deep carious lesions. Not only do MITs exhibit higher success rates compared to CT, but they also offer multiple advantages to both professionals and patients. On one hand, MITs are less traumatic for the patient, preserving more hard tissue and maintaining pulp vitality. By avoiding endodontic treatment, our restorations become easier to perform and may have a longer lifespan when performed correctly. Additionally, in most cases, we can reduce the number of appointments and the overall duration of the treatment.

Another important factor to take into account is that the follow-up period in the studies is relatively short. Most studies have a follow-up period of 1 to 3 years, while only two articles have a follow-up of 5 years [40,44]. Therefore, it would be desirable to have more long-term investigations to compare success rates. Fortunately, there are some long-term studies that are currently underway and are expected to yield new and interesting results about minimally invasive procedures [50,51]. We anticipate incorporating these investigations into future analyses. After performing Mann–Whitney U to compare mean values between MIT and CT success rate, the results showed that there was not a statistically significant difference between these variables (p-value > 0.05).

Regarding pulp exposure percentages, minimally invasive techniques present a lower incidence of this complication compared to conventional procedures. It is conceivable that conventional techniques result in greater tissue removal. As a result, it is more probable that they will harm the dental pulp and compromise the success of our restorations. In our opinion, pulp exposure is a crucial aspect to consider when treating deep carious lesions. This characteristic should be assessed in every study to demonstrate the level of conservatism of a caries removal technique. New research should focus on the frequency of treatments leading to pulp exposure and establish a comparison between procedures. Unfortunately, only four out of the seven articles included in this meta-analysis reported rates of pulp exposure. [41–43,45]. While MIT presents 1.2% of pulp exposure, this value in CT is 8.1%; almost seven times higher than the previous one.

An important aspect that we needed to consider in our investigation was whether the rates of pulp exposure were influenced by the type of procedure used for caries removal. So, we analyzed both variables statistically using Wilcoxon non-parametric test, due to the small sample of this investigation. The results of this analysis showed that there was no significant difference between both techniques (p-value > 0.05) and therefore, pulp exposure was not influenced by the kind of procedure. However, the p-value is very close to our limit of significance (p-value = 0.068), and since our sample size is very small, it is acceptable to assume that if we could have included more studies in our meta-analysis, the difference could have been significant.

The current trend in dentistry is to orient our treatments in the most conservative way. Other areas, such as surgery or prosthesis, present new minimally invasive techniques that reduce trauma to the patient, as well as the duration of treatment. However, when it comes to caries removal, in most cases, a conventional treatment protocol is still implemented, consisting of eliminating all carious tissue without respecting pulp vitality. Minimally invasive caries removal techniques, such as selective treatments, are a great alternative to complete removal procedures, showing good results in success rates of restorations and pulp exposure rates. Adapting our restorative protocols to selective caries removal techniques allows us to offer significant benefits to patients without increasing the risks or economic and time costs. With regard to the materials needed to perform minimally invasive techniques, caries detector dyes and fluorescence devices are utilized for delineating the boundaries of our restorations, facilitating the establishment of a proper peripheral seal and ensuring correct bonding. However, these materials are not always precise, and often result in excessive tissue removal and overpreparation. Therefore, new techniques and devices should be designed to be as respectful and minimally invasive as possible [11,29,30]. If we are very careful with our bonding protocol and follow selective removal procedures, we can preserve affected dentin at the pulpal wall, controlling the progression of caries. After restorative procedure, It is important to maintain a close follow-up to observe how pulp tissue responds to minimally invasive techniques while measuring pulp vitality.

In our opinion, selective removal procedures should be further investigated with larger samples in multicentric and long-term studies to obtain a gold-standard treatment protocol that could be as respectful as possible to pulp tissues, as well as very conservative with hard tissues. This way, with reliable and reproducible results, professionals worldwide can opt for selective procedures rather than conventional ones.

5. Conclusions

1. Using minimally invasive techniques for caries removal presents slightly better success results than conventional techniques, although this difference is not significant.
2. Minimally invasive techniques result in a lower percentage of pulp exposure than conventional ones, which may lead to improved success rates in those techniques.
3. More long-term RCTs in the permanent dentition are required to demonstrate whether there is a significantly reduced risk of pulp exposure and higher success in preserving pulp vitality when minimal invasive caries removal techniques are applied.

Author Contributions: Data curation, D.G.-G.; formal analysis, D.G.-G. investigation, D.G.-G., J.F.-F., V.V.-R., A.M.-V. and J.L.-M.; methodology, D.G.-G., V.V.-R., A.M.-V., J.F.-F. and J.L.-M.; project administration, D.G.-G., J.F.-F. and J.L.-M.; resources, D.G.-G., V.V.-R., A.M.-V., J.F.-F. and J.L.-M.; software, D.G.-G. and J.F.-F.; supervision, J.F.-F. and J.L.-M.; validation, J.F.-F. and J.L.-M.; visualization, D.G.-G., V.V.-R., A.M.-V. and J.L.-M.; writing—original draft, D.G.-G.; writing—review and editing, D.G.-G. and J.F.-F. All authors have read and agreed to the published version of the manuscript.

Funding: This research received no external funding.

Institutional Review Board Statement: Not applicable.

Informed Consent Statement: Not applicable.

Data Availability Statement: Data are contained within the article.

Conflicts of Interest: The authors declare they have no potential conflict of interest with respect to the re-search, authorship, and/or publication of this article.

References

1. Machiulskiene, V.; Campus, G.; Carvalho, J.C.; Dige, I.; Ekstrand, K.R.; Jablonski-Momeni, A.; Maltz, M.; Manton, D.J.; Martignon, S.; Martinez-Mier, E.A.; et al. Terminology of Dental Caries and Dental Caries Management: Consensus Report of a Workshop Organized by ORCA and Cariology Research Group of IADR. *Caries Res.* **2020**, *54*, 7–14. [CrossRef]
2. Elgezawi, M.; Haridy, R.; Abdalla, M.A.; Heck, K.; Draenert, M.; Kaisarly, D. Current Strategies to Control Recurrent and Residual Caries with Resin Composite Restorations: Operator- and Material-Related Factors. *J. Clin. Med.* **2022**, *11*, 6591. [CrossRef]
3. Leal, S.C.; Dame-Teixeira, N.; Barbosa, C.B.; Kominami, P.A.A.; Raposo, F.; Nakagawa, E.M.T.; Banerjee, A. Minimum intervention oral care: Defining the future of caries management. *Braz. Oral Res.* **2022**, *36*, e135. [CrossRef] [PubMed]
4. Jakovljevic, A.; Jaćimović, J.; Aminoshariae, A.; Fransson, H. Effectiveness of vital pulp treatment in managing nontraumatic pulpitis associated with no or nonspontaneous pain: A systematic review. *Int. Endod. J.* **2022**, *56*, 340–354. [CrossRef]
5. Schwendicke, F.; Walsh, T.; Lamont, T.; Al-Yaseen, W.; Bjørndal, L.; Clarkson, J.E.; Fontana, M.; Gomez Rossi, J.; Göstemeyer, G.; Levey, C.; et al. Interventions for treating cavitated or dentine carious lesions. *Cochrane Database Syst. Rev.* **2021**, *7*, CD013039. [CrossRef] [PubMed]
6. Barros, M.M.A.F.; De Queiroz Rodrigues, M.I.; Muniz, F.W.M.G.; Rodrigues, L.K.A. Selective, stepwise, or nonselective removal of carious tissue: Which technique offers lower risk for the treatment of dental caries in permanent teeth? A systematic review and meta-analysis. *Clin. Oral Investig.* **2020**, *24*, 521–532. [CrossRef]
7. Senthilkumar, V.; Ramesh, S. Systematic review on alternative methods for caries removal in permanent teeth. *J. Conserv. Dent.* **2020**, *23*, 2–9. [CrossRef]
8. Ferreira Zandona, A.G. Surgical Management of Caries Lesions: Selective Removal of Carious Tissues. *Dent. Clin. North. Am.* **2019**, *63*, 705–713. [CrossRef]
9. Ricketts, D.; Lamont, T.; Innes, N.P.; Kidd, E.; Clarkson, J.E. Operative caries management in adults and children. *Cochrane Database Syst. Rev.* **2019**, *7*, CD003808. [CrossRef]
10. Ricketts, D.; Innes, N.; Schwendicke, F. Selective Removal of Carious Tissue. *Monogr. Oral Sci.* **2018**, *27*, 82–91. [CrossRef]
11. Alleman, D.S.; Magne, P. A systematic approach to deep caries removal end points: The peripheral seal concept in adhesive dentistry. *Quintessence Int.* **2012**, *43*, 197–208. [PubMed]
12. Jurasic, M.M.; Gillespie, S.; Sorbara, P.; Clarkson, J.; Ramsay, C.; Nyongesa, D.; McEdward, D.; Gilbert, G.H.; Vollmer, W.M.; National Dental PBRN Collaborative Group. Deep caries removal strategies: Findings from The National Dental Practice-Based Research Network. *J. Am. Dent. Assoc.* **2022**, *153*, 1078–1088.e7. [CrossRef] [PubMed]
13. Bjørndal, L.; Simon, S.; Tomson, P.L.; Duncan, H.F. Management of deep caries and the exposed pulp. *Int. Endod. J.* **2019**, *52*, 949–973. [CrossRef] [PubMed]
14. Faria, L.V.; Fernandes, T.O.; Guimarães, L.S.; Cajazeira, M.R.R.; Antunes, L.S.; Antunes, L.A.A. Does selective caries removal in combination with antimicrobial photodynamic therapy affect the clinical performance of adhesive restorations of primary or permanent teeth? A systematic review with meta-analysis. *J. Clin. Pediatr. Dent.* **2022**, *46*, 1–14. [CrossRef] [PubMed]

15. Li, T.; Zhai, X.; Song, F.; Zhu, H. Selective versus non-selective removal for dental caries: A systematic review and meta-analysis. *Acta Odontol. Scand.* **2018**, *76*, 135–140. [CrossRef] [PubMed]
16. Schwendicke, F. Contemporary concepts in carious tissue removal: A review. *J. Esthet. Restor. Dent.* **2017**, *29*, 403–408. [CrossRef]
17. Schwendicke, F.; Göstemeyer, G. Understanding dentists' management of deep carious lesions in permanent teeth: A systematic review and meta-analysis. *Implement. Sci.* **2016**, *11*, 142. [CrossRef]
18. Dorri, M.; Martinez-Zapata, M.J.; Walsh, T.; Marinho, V.C.; Sheiham Deceased, A.; Zaror, C. Atraumatic restorative treatment versus conventional restorative treatment for managing dental caries. *Cochrane Database Syst. Rev.* **2017**, *12*, CD008072. [CrossRef]
19. Hoefler, V.; Nagaoka, H.; Miller, C.S. Long-term survival and vitality outcomes of permanent teeth following deep caries treatment with step-wise and partial-caries-removal: A Systematic Review. *J. Dent.* **2016**, *54*, 25–32. [CrossRef]
20. Banerjee, A. "MI" caries management--an overview. *Ann. R. Australas. Coll. Dent. Surg.* **2012**, *21*, 43–48.
21. Thompson, V.; Craig, R.G.; Curro, F.A.; Green, W.S.; Ship, J.A. Treatment of deep carious lesions by complete excavation or partial removal: A critical review. *J. Am. Dent. Assoc.* **2008**, *139*, 705–712. [CrossRef] [PubMed]
22. Perić, T.; Marković, D.; Zivković, S. Dental caries--therapeutic possibilities. *Srp. Arh. Celok. Lek.* **2008**, *136*, 662–666. [CrossRef] [PubMed]
23. Sadasiva, K.; Kumar, K.S.; Rayar, S.; Shamini, S.; Unnikrishnan, M.; Kandaswamy, D. Evaluation of the Efficacy of Visual, Tactile Method, Caries Detector Dye, and Laser Fluorescence in Removal of Dental Caries and Confirmation by Culture and Polymerase Chain Reaction: An In Vivo Study. *J. Pharm. Bioallied Sci.* **2019**, *11* (Suppl. S2), S146–S150. [CrossRef]
24. Hosoya, Y.; Taguchi, T.; Tay, F.R. Evaluation of a new caries detecting dye for primary and permanent carious dentin. *J. Dent.* **2007**, *35*, 137–143. [CrossRef]
25. Maru, V.P.; Shakuntala, B.S.; Nagarathna, C. Caries Removal by Chemomechanical (Carisolv™) vs. Rotary Drill: A Systematic Review. *Open Dent. J.* **2015**, *9*, 462–472. [CrossRef]
26. Hamama, H.H.; Yiu, C.K.; Burrow, M.F.; King, N.M. Systematic Review and Meta-Analysis of Randomized Clinical Trials on Chemomechanical Caries Removal. *Oper. Dent.* **2015**, *40*, E167–E178. [CrossRef]
27. Bratu, D.C.; Nikolajevic-Stoican, N.; Popa, G.; Pop, S.I.; Dragoș, B.; Luca, M.M. A Bibliometric Analysis (2010–2020) of the Dental Scientific Literature on Chemo-Mechanical Methods of Caries Removal Using Carisolv and BRIX3000. *Medicina* **2022**, *58*, 788. [CrossRef]
28. Hosein, T.; Hasan, A. Efficacy of chemo-mechanical caries removal with Carisolv. *J. Coll. Physicians Surg. Pak.* **2008**, *18*, 222–225.
29. Akbari, M.; Ahrari, F.; Jafari, M. A comparative evaluation of DIAGNOdent and caries detector dye in detection of residual caries in prepared cavities. *J. Contemp. Dent. Pract.* **2012**, *13*, 515–520. [CrossRef]
30. Trippe, L.H.; Ribeiro, A.A.; Azcarate-Peril, M.A.; Preisser, J.S.; Wang, R.; Zandona, A.F. Is Fluorescence Technology a Promising Tool for Detecting Infected Dentin in Deep Carious Lesions? *Caries Res.* **2020**, *54*, 205–217. [CrossRef]
31. Lennon, A.M.; Attin, T.; Martens, S.; Buchalla, W. Fluorescence-aided caries excavation (FACE), caries detector, and conventional caries excavation in primary teeth. *Pediatr. Dent.* **2009**, *31*, 316–319. [PubMed]
32. Giacaman, R.A.; Muñoz-Sandoval, C.; Neuhaus, K.W.; Fontana, M.; Chałas, R. Evidence-based strategies for the minimally invasive treatment of carious lesions: Review of the literature. *Adv. Clin. Exp. Med.* **2018**, *27*, 1009–1016. [CrossRef] [PubMed]
33. Schwendicke, F.; Frencken, J.E.; Bjørndal, L.; Maltz, M.; Manton, D.J.; Ricketts, D.; Van Landuyt, K.; Banerjee, A.; Campus, G.; Doméjean, S.; et al. Managing Carious Lesions: Consensus Recommendations on Carious Tissue Removal. *Adv. Dent. Res.* **2016**, *28*, 58–67. [CrossRef] [PubMed]
34. Alsadat, F.A.; El-Housseiny, A.A.; Alamoudi, N.M.; Alnowaiser, A.M. Conservative treatment for deep carious lesions in primary and young permanent teeth. *Niger. J. Clin. Pract.* **2018**, *21*, 1549–1556. [CrossRef]
35. Hassan, A.F.; Yadav, G.; Tripathi, A.M.; Mehrotra, M.; Saha, S.; Garg, N. A Comparative Evaluation of the Efficacy of Different Caries Excavation Techniques in reducing the Cariogenic Flora: An in vivo Study. *Int. J. Clin. Pediatr. Dent.* **2016**, *9*, 214–217. [CrossRef] [PubMed]
36. Tjäderhane, L.; Tezvergil-Mutluay, A. Performance of Adhesives and Restorative Materials After Selective Removal of Carious Lesions: Restorative Materials with Anticaries Properties. *Dent. Clin. N. Am.* **2019**, *63*, 715–729. [CrossRef] [PubMed]
37. de Almeida Neves, A.; Coutinho, E.; Cardoso, M.V.; Lambrechts, P.; Van Meerbeek, B. Current concepts and techniques for caries excavation and adhesion to residual dentin. *J. Adhes. Dent.* **2011**, *13*, 7–22. [CrossRef] [PubMed]
38. Isolan, C.P.; Sarkis-Onofre, R.; Lima, G.S.; Moraes, R.R. Bonding to Sound and Caries-Affected Dentin: A Systematic Review and Meta-Analysis. *J. Adhes. Dent.* **2018**, *20*, 7–18. [CrossRef]
39. Gözetici-Çil, B.; Erdem-Hepşenoğlu, Y.; Tekin, A.; Özcan, M. Selective removal to soft dentine or selective removal to firm dentine for deep caries lesions in permanent posterior teeth: A randomized controlled clinical trial up to 2 years. *Clin. Oral Investig.* **2022**, 1–13. [CrossRef]
40. Jardim, J.J.; Mestrinho, H.D.; Koppe, B.; de Paula, L.M.; Alves, L.S.; Yamaguti, P.M.; Almeida, J.C.F.; Maltz, M. Restorations after selective caries removal: 5-Year randomized trial. *J. Dent.* **2020**, *99*, 103416. [CrossRef]
41. Labib, M.E.; Hassanein, O.E.; Moussa, M.; Yassen, A.; Schwendicke, F. Selective versus stepwise removal of deep carious lesions in permanent teeth: A randomised controlled trial from Egypt-an interim analysis. *BMJ Open* **2019**, *9*, e030957. [CrossRef] [PubMed]
42. Ali, A.H.; Koller, G.; Foschi, F.; Andiappan, M.; Bruce, K.D.; Banerjee, A.; Mannocci, F. Self-Limiting versus Conventional Caries Removal: A Randomized Clinical Trial. *J. Dent. Res.* **2018**, *97*, 1207–1213. [CrossRef] [PubMed]

43. Khokhar, M.; Tewari, S. Outcomes of Partial and Complete Caries Excavation in Permanent Teeth: A 18 Month Clinical Study. *Contemp. Clin. Dent.* **2018**, *9*, 468–473. [CrossRef] [PubMed]
44. Maltz, M.; Koppe, B.; Jardim, J.J.; Alves, L.S.; de Paula, L.M.; Yamaguti, P.M.; Almeida, J.C.F.; Moura, M.S.; Mestrinho, H.D. Partial caries removal in deep caries lesions: A 5-year multicenter randomized controlled trial. *Clin. Oral Investig.* **2018**, *22*, 1337–1343. [CrossRef] [PubMed]
45. Casagrande, L.; Seminario, A.T.; Correa, M.B.; Werle, S.B.; Maltz, M.; Demarco, F.F.; Araujo, F.B. Longevity and associated risk factors in adhesive restorations of young permanent teeth after complete and selective caries removal: A retrospective study. *Clin. Oral Investig.* **2017**, *21*, 847–855. [CrossRef]
46. Faria, L.V.; Antunes, L.S.; Pio, L.R.R.; Dias, J.C.; Pinheiro, L.H.M.; Reis, C.L.B.; Fontes, K.B.F.C.; Cajazeira, M.R.R.; Antunes, L.A.A. Evaluation of composite restorations in primary molars subjected to selective caries removal associated with antimicrobial photodynamic therapy: A randomized controlled trial. *Int. J. Paediatr. Dent.* **2022**, *32*, 585–597. [CrossRef]
47. Elhennawy, K.; Finke, C.; Paris, S.; Reda, S.; Jost-Brinkmann, P.G.; Schwendicke, F. Selective vs stepwise removal of deep carious lesions in primary molars: 24 months follow-up from a randomized controlled trial. *Clin. Oral Investig.* **2021**, *25*, 645–652. [CrossRef]
48. Liberman, J.; Franzon, R.; Guimarães, L.F.; Casagrande, L.; Haas, A.N.; Araujo, F.B. Survival of composite restorations after selective or total caries removal in primary teeth and predictors of failures: A 36-months randomized controlled trial. *J. Dent.* **2020**, *93*, 103268. [CrossRef]
49. Kochhar, G.K.; Srivastava, N.; Pandit, I.K.; Gugnani, N.; Gupta, M. An evaluation of different caries removal techniques in primary teeth: A comparitive clinical study. *J. Clin. Pediatr. Dent.* **2011**, *36*, 5–9. [CrossRef]
50. Clarkson, J.E.; Ramsay, C.R.; Ricketts, D.; Banerjee, A.; Deery, C.; Lamont, T.; Boyers, D.; Marshman, Z.; Goulao, B.; Banister, K.; et al. Selective Caries Removal in Permanent Teeth (SCRiPT) for the treatment of deep carious lesions: A randomised controlled clinical trial in primary care. *BMC Oral Health* **2021**, *21*, 336. [CrossRef] [PubMed]
51. Schwendicke, F.; Leal, S.; Schlattmann, P.; Paris, S.; Dias Ribeiro, A.P.; Gomes Marques, M.; Hilgert, L.A. Selective carious tissue removal using subjective criteria or polymer bur: Study protocol for a randomised controlled trial (SelecCT). *BMJ Open* **2018**, *8*, e022952. [CrossRef] [PubMed]

Disclaimer/Publisher's Note: The statements, opinions and data contained in all publications are solely those of the individual author(s) and contributor(s) and not of MDPI and/or the editor(s). MDPI and/or the editor(s) disclaim responsibility for any injury to people or property resulting from any ideas, methods, instructions or products referred to in the content.

Article

Clinical Investigation of the Inhibitory Effects of Tooth-Coating Materials on Initial Active Root Caries: A Pilot Randomized Controlled Trial

Yoko Asahi [1,*], Katsuaki Naito [1], Hikaru Kanda [1], Kazuaki Niwano [2], Daisuke Takegawa [3], Hiromichi Yumoto [4], Yuichiro Noiri [2] and Mikako Hayashi [1]

1. Department of Restorative Dentistry and Endodontology, Osaka University Graduate School of Dentistry, Osaka 565-0871, Japan; naito.katsuaki.dent@osaka-u.ac.jp (K.N.); kanda-hikaru@dent.osaka-u.ac.jp (H.K.); hayashi.mikako.dent@osaka-u.ac.jp (M.H.)
2. Division of Cariology, Operative Dentistry and Endodontics, Department of Oral Health Science, Niigata University Graduate School of Medical and Dental Sciences, Niigata 951-8514, Japan; niwano@dent.niigata-u.ac.jp (K.N.); noiri@dent.niigata-u.ac.jp (Y.N.)
3. Department of Regenerative Dental Medicine, Tokushima University Graduate School of Biomedical Sciences, Tokushima 770-8504, Japan; d-takegawa@tokushima-u.ac.jp
4. Department of Periodontology and Endodontology, Tokushima University Graduate School of Biomedical Sciences, Tokushima 770-8504, Japan; yumoto@tokushima-u.ac.jp
* Correspondence: asahi.yoko.dent@osaka-u.ac.jp; Tel.: +81-6-6879-2927

Abstract: *Background and Objectives*: Caredyne ZIF-C is a novel, capsule-mixed zinc-containing prototype glass ionomer cement (GIC). Zinc ions are reported to inhibit root dentin demineralization, dentin collagen degradation, bacterial growth, acid production, and in vitro bacterial biofilm formation. However, the effectiveness of GICs against initial root caries lesions is unclear. Therefore, this study aimed to evaluate the efficacy of GICs, especially the new zinc-containing Caredyne ZIF-C GIC, as tooth-coating materials in patients with initial active root caries. *Materials and Methods*: A total of 58 lesions in 47 older adults (age > 65 years) were randomly allocated to one of the following three groups: Caredyne ZIF-C, Fuji VII (a conventional GIC), and sodium fluoride (NaF). All the lesions were treated with the assigned materials without removing the infected dentin, and the rates of dental plaque attachment and coating material fall-out were evaluated after 3, 6, and 12 months. The failure rate was defined as the number of teeth that needed restoration due to caries progression. *Results*: The plaque attachment rates tended to be lower in the material-coated root surfaces than in the healthy exposed root surfaces after 3, 6, and 12 months, although the differences among the three groups were not significant. Moreover, the coating material fall-out rate tended to be lower in the Caredyne ZIF-C group than in the Fuji VII group. There was no significant difference in the failure rate among the three groups at the 12 months mark. *Conclusions*: Though this pilot study offers a new direction for suppressing the progression of initial active root caries by controlling plaque attachment using GICs including Caredyne ZIF-C, clinical studies with a larger sample size are needed.

Keywords: root caries; secondary prevention; glass ionomer cement; Caredyne ZIF-C; biofilm

1. Introduction

The worldwide increase in life expectancy and advances in dental care have led to the increased retention of teeth in older individuals. However, the prevalence of gingival recession increases with age; therefore, the incidence and prevalence of root caries in this population have also increased, currently posing a significant problem worldwide [1,2]. Root surface dentin has a critical pH of <6.4, which is higher than that of enamel (<5.5), as well as a lower mineral content than that of enamel, making it more susceptible to caries [3]. Additionally, it is difficult to determine the range of repair treatment for initial root caries because the margins of the lesion are unclear, and the removal or repair of the lesion is challenging in many cases. Moreover, teeth damaged by root caries often need to be extracted, resulting in reduced oral function. Therefore, demineralization and formation of new root caries lesions should be prevented by improving the acid resistance of root surfaces susceptible to caries.

For initial demineralized lesions, a non-invasive treatment to inhibit caries progression and achieve the remineralization of the infected root dentin without "drilling and filling" is considered more beneficial for patients [4,5]. Several approaches have been proposed for inactivating root caries lesions, most of which involve the use of fluoride. In the literature review by Gluzman et al. [6], the recommendations for secondary prevention of root caries in the general adult population and vulnerable older individuals are the daily usage of a 4500–5000 ppm sodium fluoride (NaF) toothpaste gel as self-care and the application of 22,500 ppm NaF varnish every 1–3 months as professional care. According to the meta-analysis by Wierichs et al., dentifrices containing 5000 ppm fluoride or 1450 ppm fluoride with 1.5% arginine were more effective at inactivating root caries lesions (inactivating 51% more root caries lesions with 5000 ppm fluoride and 21% with 1450 ppm fluoride with 1.5% arginine) than dentifrices containing 1100–1450 ppm fluoride [7]. Another meta-analysis reported that, compared with no treatment, the use of a 38% silver diamine fluoride solution alone or with potassium iodide applied annually, 5% NaF varnish, or 1% chlorhexidine with 1% thymol varnish was associated with a two to three times greater chance of arresting or reversing root surface lesions, although the certainty of the evidence was very low [8].

In contrast, only few clinical studies have investigated the efficacy of tooth surface-coating materials in the secondary prevention of the demineralization of root caries lesions, although the dentin adhesives used as sealants in these studies have shown promising results in preventing further demineralization [9,10]. A few in vitro studies investigating the efficacy of dentin sealants in preventing root caries have claimed that dentin bonding can stabilize caries-affected areas by protecting the exposed surfaces and preventing the progression of demineralization [11,12]. Though bonding sealant acts as only a physical barrier shielding the lesion from further acid attacks, it could serve as an alternative approach for patients with initial root caries who have difficulty in receiving frequent professional care involving fluoride application or self-care with high-concentration fluoride dentifrices.

Glass ionomer cements (GICs) have been used as restorative materials. GICs are commonly used in the treatment of advanced root caries [13,14], as these have proven useful in cases of the extension of caries to the subgingival area or when moisture control is difficult [4]. GICs adhere to the tooth surface directly and release fluoride, which inhibits bacterial growth and enhances tooth structure by forming fluorapatite [15]. Remineralization can occur owing to changes in environmental conditions that spread within the dental biofilm-covered carious lesions [16]. Thus, controlling and inhibiting dental biofilm formation or the application of materials that have an effect on hardening dentine could inhibit demineralization and promote remineralization. An in vitro study using a bovine carious dentin model showed that both conventional GIC and a mineral trioxide aggregate induced mineral density gain [17]. In previous clinical studies, GIC sealants were shown to be effective in reducing the progression of initial enamel proximal caries [18] or arresting microcavitated (ICDAS 3) coronal carious lesions [19]. Therefore, the application of GICs as a coating material is expected to inhibit dental biofilm formation and surface root caries progression, and its effectiveness is expected to be higher than that of resin bonding, which is another candidate coating material which has no antibacterial or remineralization effects.

Caredyne ZIF-C (GC Dental Industrial Corporation, Tokyo, Japan) is a novel capsule-mixed zinc-containing prototype GIC, which is a commercially available variant of GIC Caredyne Restore; it contains a BioUnion filler [20] and releases calcium, fluoride, and zinc ions. Reportedly, zinc ions can inhibit root dentin demineralization, dentin collagen degradation, bacterial growth, acid production, and biofilm formation in vitro [21–27]. Using GICs as coating materials for initial active root caries not only physically protects carious lesions but is also expected to suppress root caries progression through their anti-biofilm effects and improvement of dentine structure through the incorporation of fluoride.

Caredyne ZIF-C would have an especially strong effect as it contains zinc in addition to fluoride. However, to the best of our knowledge, no clinical study has reported on the use of GICs as coating materials for the management of initial root caries; therefore, the effect of GICs against plaque attachment, caries progression, or remineralization of initial root caries lesions is unclear. Thus, our research objective was to assess the extent of stabilization of root caries lesions with GICs as the tooth-coating materials. Focusing on the regulation of biofilm formation, the aim of this study was to evaluate the effects of Caredyne ZIF-C and a conventional GIC (Fuji VII Capsule; GC Dental Industrial Corporation, Tokyo, Japan) on dental biofilm attachment on initial active root caries, in comparison to a NaF solution. Moreover, we assessed the failure rate, which was defined as the need for restoration due to caries progression. The NaF solution was selected as the target for comparison because it is commonly used in Japan. We hypothesized that Caredyne ZIF-C, which contains zinc in addition to fluoride and inhibits biofilm formation more significantly than Fuji VII in vitro [21], would have the highest plaque attachment inhibitory effect; we conducted a pilot randomized controlled trial that included 18 teeth in each group.

2. Materials and Methods

2.1. Study Design

This pilot randomized controlled trial was conducted at three universities in Japan using a parallel-group design. The study protocol was reviewed and approved by the Ethics Committee of the Osaka University Graduate School of Dentistry (H30-E40-3), the Ethics Committee of Niigata University (Approval number 2019-0007), and the Ethics Committee of Tokushima University Hospital (3573-3) and was registered prior to participant recruitment with the University Hospital Medical Information Network-Clinical Trial Registry (UMIN-CTR; No. UMIN000035609, registered on 22 January 2019).

2.2. Recruitment

Older patients (age > 65 years) were recruited at three university hospitals: Osaka University Dental Hospital, Niigata University Medical and Dental Hospital, and Tokushima University Hospital. The inclusion criterion was the presence of at least one permanent tooth with initial active root caries lesions, specifically those classified as code 1 of the International Caries Detection and Assessment System (ICDAS II) classification [28] and soft/leathery lesions. Patients with advanced root caries that needed drilling and those who could not visit the hospital every 3 months were excluded from this study. The informed consent form was explained to and read by the patients, and written informed consent was obtained from all the participants prior to clinical examinations.

2.3. Baseline Examinations

Clinical examinations were performed, and information regarding the number of remaining teeth, the decayed, missing, and filled teeth score, and the plaque control record was obtained. The root caries lesions were also assessed by means of a visual and tactile examination to evaluate the color (yellow/light brown/dark brown/black) and hardness (soft/leathery). Saliva was stimulated using a gum provided in the kit and was collected to calculate the salivary flow rate and the salivary bacterial counts. The Saliva-Check LAB® (GC Dental Industrial Corporation, Tokyo, Japan) was used according to the manufacturer's instructions to estimate streptococci, mutans streptococci, and lactobacilli counts using a real-time polymerase chain reaction, as previously reported [29].

2.4. Randomized Allocation

An independent researcher performed randomization using a random number table. The original random allocation sequence was maintained at a separate location. The patients were randomly allocated in a double-blind manner to one of the following three treatment groups: Caredyne, FUJI VII, and NaF. If a patient had multiple teeth with root caries lesions, more than two teeth per patient were included in the study; however, the same treatment method was applied to all teeth in an oral cavity.

2.5. Interventions

The tooth-coating materials used in this study (two sealants and one fluoride solution) are shown in Table 1.

Table 1. Tooth-coating materials used in this study.

Material	Composition	Manufacturer
Caredyne ZIF-C	Powder: fluoroaluminosilicate glass, fluorozincsilicate glass (BioUnion filler), polyacrylic acid Liquid: polyacrylic acid, distilled water, polybasic carboxylic acid, phosphoric acid	GC Dental Industrial Corporation, Tokyo, Japan
FUJI VII capsule	Powder: fluoroaluminosilicate glass Liquid: polyacrylic acid, distilled water, polybasic carboxylic acid	GC Dental Industrial Corporation, Tokyo, Japan
Sodium fluoride solution 2%	2% acidulated phosphate sodium fluoride	BEE BRAND MEDICO DENTAL. CO., LTD, Osaka, Japan

The target teeth were professionally cleaned and isolated using cotton rolls; the saliva was removed using a cotton pellet, and the teeth were dried using a three-way syringe. The allocated material was then applied without removing the carious dentin. The fluoride solution was applied for 4 min. For the sealants, the tooth surface was first treated with a cavity conditioner for 10 s and then washed and dried. The sealants were mechanically mixed for 10 s (Capsule Mixer CM-II; GC Dental Industrial Corporation, Tokyo, Japan), applied to the root surface, and coated with varnish.

2.6. Follow-Up Examinations

Follow-up examinations were conducted at 3, 6, and 12 months after the baseline by the same examiner. The color and texture of the lesions and the adhesion of the sealants were evaluated via an inspection. The hardness of the lesions was estimated by means of palpation using a Community Periodontal Index (CPI) probe [30,31]. The color and hardness of the lesions and the degree of demineralization in the GIC groups were evaluated to the extent possible, even in cases wherein the coating material was detached. The rate of attachment of dental plaque was assessed based on oral photographs obtained after staining the plaque with Butler GUM RED-COTE (Sunstar, Osaka, Japan). The root surface area and plaque attachment area on the oral photographs were measured using a polygon selections tool in an image analysis software (ImageJ version 1.53; NIH, Bethesda, MD, USA), and the residual rate of plaque on the root surface was calculated. Healthy exposed root surfaces in each participant were used as the control. We selected the same type of tooth as the coated tooth to the extent possible in the following priority order: adjacent tooth, opposite tooth, and opposing tooth. The image analysis was performed by an independent researcher who was blinded to the treatment groups, and the data were encoded. The failure rate was calculated by the number of teeth that needed restoration due to caries progression. The fluoride solution in the NaF group was applied every 3 months, whereas the GIC sealants in the Caredyne ZIF-C and Fuji VII groups were re-applied only if a partial or complete loss of the sealant was noted. Calibration was performed before the start of the trial to ensure the uniformity of the assessment methods and techniques.

2.7. Sample Size

No previous clinical studies were available for reference regarding sample size calculation; therefore, a minimum of 15 teeth were estimated to be required in each group [32]. Assuming a 15% dropout rate, 18 teeth were included in each group in this study.

2.8. Statistical Analysis

All statistical analyses were performed using SPSS ver. 22.0 (IBM SPSS Inc., Armonk, NY, USA). This study was conducted under the intention-to-treat principle. Fisher's exact test was used to analyze the sealant material fall-out rate, the failure rate, the baseline characteristics of the teeth, and potential sex differences. The Kruskal–Wallis test was used to assess the residual rate of dental plaque and compare the patient characteristics at the baseline. Spearman's rank correlation coefficient analysis was used to assess the correlation between salivary flow and dental plaque accumulation. The level of statistical significance was set to 5%.

3. Results

Fifty-one older adults (65 teeth) underwent dental examinations at the three university hospitals between April 2019 and April 2022, and 47 individuals (58 teeth) who met the eligibility criteria and agreed to participate were enrolled in this study. After 3, 6, and 12 months, the dropout rates were, respectively, as follows: 11.1%, 11.1%, and 22% in the Caredyne ZIF-C group; 0%, 4.5%, and 31.8% in the Fuji VII group; and 0%, 11.1%, and 22% in the NaF group (Figure 1).

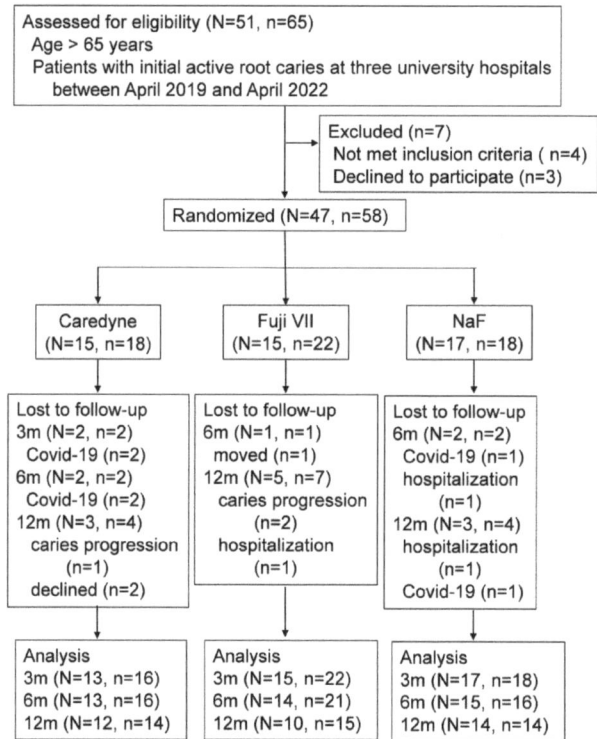

Figure 1. Flowchart of the study participants. N = participants with root caries, n = root caries lesions.

The main reasons for dropout were related to hospitalization and COVID-19.

Table 2 presents the baseline demographic characteristics of the study participants; no statistically significant differences were observed among the three groups in terms of any of these variables.

Table 2. Baseline demographic characteristics of the participants.

	Caredyne	Fuji VII	NaF	p-Value
Mean age (SD)	72 (5.5)	75 (6.2)	73 (6.4)	0.26
Sex				0.13
Male	7 (47%)	9 (60%)	4 (23.5%)	
Female	8 (53%)	6 (40%)	13 (76.5%)	
Mean number of remaining teeth (range)	24 (19–29)	20 (4–29)	24 (17–28)	0.26
DMFT (SD)	18.9 (6.9)	20.9 (4.6)	17.6 (5.8)	0.29
PCR (SD)	31.6 (12.8)	44.5 (17.8)	33.4 (16.5)	0.1
Salivary flow rate (mL/min)				
Mean (SD)	1.37 (0.60)	1.04 (0.67)	1.03 (0.51)	0.19
≤1.0 mL/min (%)	33.3	53.3	52.9	0.28
>1.0 mL/min (%)	66.7	46.7	47.1	0.35
Salivary bacterial count				
Streptococci (10^7/mL)	6.69	8.83	3.9	0.06
Mutans streptococci				
S. mutans (10^4/mL)	2.7	6.1	3.6	0.11
S. sobrinus (10^5/mL)	0.4	10.3	1.7	0.18
Lactobacillus (10^7/mL)	1	13.8	5.3	0.25

Table 3 shows the distribution of tooth types and affected sites, which were scattered among the three groups.

Table 3. Distribution of the tooth types included in this study.

Tooth	Caredyne	Fuji VII	NaF
Maxilla			
Incisor	4 (2)	2 (2)	8 (6)
Canine	2(2)	2 (1)	1 (1)
Premolar	5 (4)	3 (1)	1
Molar	3 (3)	1	3 (2)
Mandible			
Incisor	0	2 (2)	2 (1)
Canine	1	6 (3)	0
Premolar	3 (1)	6 (4)	3 (3)
Molar	0	0	0

Parentheses indicate values for the teeth on the right side.

The baseline characteristics of the root caries lesions are presented in Table 4; no statistically significant differences in color, texture, or hardness were observed.

Table 4. Baseline characteristics of the teeth.

	Caredyne	Fuji VII	NaF
Color			
Pale yellow			1
Light brown	10	9	8
Dark brown	6	6	4
Black	2	7	5
Hardness			
Soft	2	5	1
Leathery	16	17	17

Figure 2 shows the fall-out rates of the Caredyne ZIF-C and Fuji VII coating materials.

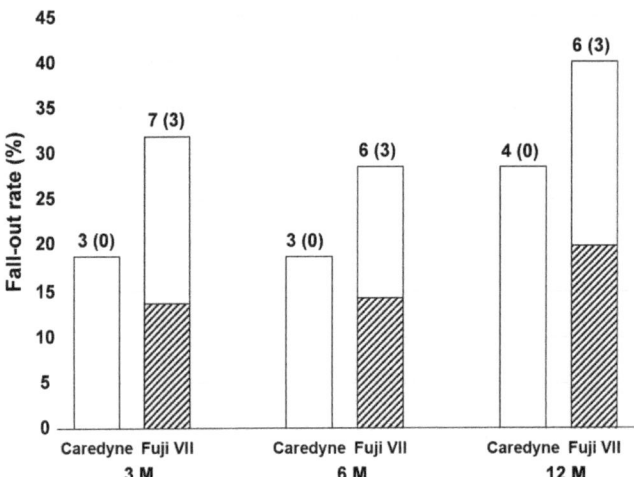

Figure 2. Fall-out rate of the coating materials. The hatched bar indicates partial defects. The numbers above the bar indicate the sample size. Parentheses indicate partial defects. Fisher's exact test, $p > 0.05$.

Although the material fall-out rate tended to be higher in the Fuji VII group, the difference was not significant. The rate of partial loss of the material was higher in the Fuji VII group than in the Caredyne ZIF-C group. The fall-out of material was not found to be associated with lesions' surface hardness or tooth type (Table S1). The detachment of materials occurred more frequently on the defect side of the clasped tooth. Among the lesions with fall-out, some had improved lesion texture, from rough to smooth, and lesion hardness, from soft/leathery to hard, while others showed caries progression and needed drilling and filling.

The outcomes related to the attachment rate of dental plaque are presented in Figure 3.

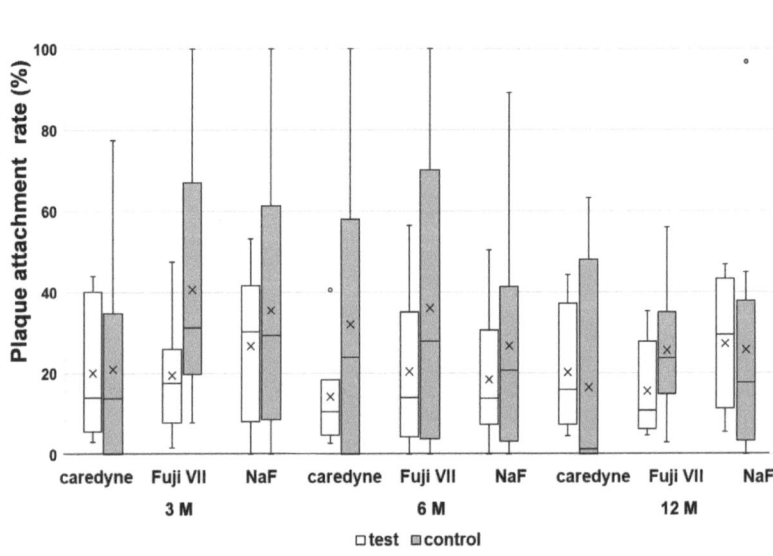

Figure 3. Rate of dental plaque attachment. "Test" indicates material-coated root surfaces, and "control" indicates healthy exposed root surfaces. Circles represent outliers. "X" indicates the mean. Kruskal–Wallis test, $p > 0.05$.

Although the Kruskal–Wallis test did not reveal any significant differences among the three groups in the rate of dental plaque attachment at 3, 6, and 12 months, the rates tended to decrease in the treatment groups. There were no strong correlations between the salivary flow rate and the rate of dental plaque attachment (3 months: $rs = -0.027$; 6 months: $rs = -0.104$; and 12 months: $rs = -0.41$).

Between 3 and 6 months after the baseline, one patient in each of the GIC groups required restorative treatment due to the progression of root caries, resulting in failure rates of 5.88% in the Caredyne ZIF-C group and 4.65% in the FUJI VII group ($p = 0.621$). The treated teeth in both the Caredyne ZIF-C and Fuji VII groups were clasped teeth on the defect side. Between 6 and 12 months after the baseline, one patient in each group required restorative treatment due to the progression of root caries, and the failure rates were 6.25% in the Caredyne ZIF-C group, 5.4% in the FUJI VII group, and 6.25% in the NaF group ($p = 0.998$).

4. Discussion

Currently, high-concentration fluoride liquids or varnishes are used in professional care to effectively arrest root caries lesions. In this study, we aimed to stabilize the lesions by suppressing the progression of root caries as well as by physically protecting them from acid challenges in the long term. In this pilot study, the following results were obtained. There were no significant differences in the failure rates among the three groups at 12 months. Although the plaque attachment rates tended to be lower in the GICs-coated root surfaces than in the healthy exposed root surfaces, there were no significant differences. Moreover, the coating material fall-out rate tended to be lower in the Caredyne ZIF-C group than in the Fuji VII group. Although no significant differences were obtained, indicating a lack of immediate clinical application, this study demonstrated the potential for managing initial active root caries. Consequently, further clinical research in this area is warranted. While fluoride application is widely used in the management of initial root caries, the results of this study might lead to a new option for secondary prevention, which involves coating root caries lesions with bioactive materials.

The fall-out rates for the GIC coatings used in this study were higher than those in the daily treatment. In previous works, demineralization was reported to have a significant effect on the dentin bond strengths of Caredyne ZIF-C and Fuji VII, though these bond strengths were less influenced when compared to those of resin composites [33]; coating root caries lesions without the removal of carious dentin may induce a higher fall-out rate. In a study by Wicht et al., root caries lesions were sealed after the removal of the infected dentin [9], whereas, in another study by Baysan et al., root sealant was applied to the lesions without removing the carious dentin [10]. The removal of carious dentin prior to coating a lesion is expected to reduce the fall-out rates of materials, although it has not yet been established whether infected dentin should be removed or not.

The fall-out rates were approximately 20% (Caredyne ZIF-C group) and 30% (Fuji VII group) in this study after 3 months and 6 months and increased to 30% (Caredyne ZIF-C group) and 40% (Fuji VII group) after 12 months. Therefore, the recall period for a GIC-coated tooth can be considered to be 6–12 months. Hence, compared to the established fluoride treatments, the assumed interval of intervention will be longer in the GICs coating approach. Meanwhile, since there were no significant differences in the failure rate (the rate of teeth which needed restoration) after 12 months, it is indicative that coating with GICs is as cost-effective as coating with fluoride. In particular, the protection of lesions with GICs might have a potential advantage over fluoride application for patients who have difficulty in frequently visiting a dental clinic or engaging in self-care. The defect side of the clasped tooth appeared to have some difficulty retaining the coating materials; therefore, it is recommended to avoid using them on clasped teeth.

Partial defects of the coating material were observed in the Fuji VII group. Nagasawa et al. investigated the effects of saliva contamination and/or dentin demineralization on the shear bond strength between bovine root dentin and Caredyne ZIF-C, Fuji VII, and resin composites [33]. They reported that cohesive failure was common with Fuji VII regardless of the experimental conditions, although adhesive failure was also observed with Caredyne ZIF-C, especially under demineralized dentin without saliva and with severe saliva contamination. They also reported that the compressive strength, diametral tensile strength, and flexural strength of Fuji VII were lower than those of other restorative materials and that Caredyne ZIF-C was more difficult to wear and disintegrate than Fuji VII and fell out in blocks, without chipping.

We have previously reported that Caredyne Restore (GC Dental Industrial Corporation, Tokyo, Japan), a non-capsule-type Caredyne ZIF-C variant, inhibited *Streptococcus mutans* biofilm formation in vitro by interfering with bacterial adhesion more effectively than hydroxyapatite disks and FUJI VII ($p < 0.05$) [21]. Similarly, Nishida et al. reported that zinc-fluoride glass nanoparticles (Zinc-F) suppressed *S. mutans* and *Actinomyces naeslundii* biofilm formation; they hypothesized that Zinc-F had anti-biofilm effects and inhibited the growth of oral bacteria by releasing multiple ions [34]. In the present study, although the dental plaque attachment rate showed a downward trend, a significant difference was not observed, unlike what had been expected. While the above in vitro studies evaluated anti-biofilm effects after 24 h of incubation, we evaluated the residual dental biofilm 3 months after professional cleaning, and biofilm maturation in this context might be different from that observed in vitro, which may have led to non-significant results. To investigate the effects of tooth-coating materials on bacterial adhesion, it is necessary to evaluate them over a shorter period of time. Notably, Caredyne Restore was found to reduce biofilm thickness and the ratio of live/dead bacteria in vitro [35]. It would be interesting to clarify the multi-faceted effects of these tooth-coating materials on oral cavity biofilms. Another potential reason for the non-significant results is the large variation in plaque attachment rate in the controls (healthy exposed root surface) among the three groups. Therefore, we will consider comparing the plaque attachment at the baseline as well as after coating the materials on the same root surface in the future.

Kohno et al. reported that the concentration of Zn^{2+} released from a GIC-containing BioUnion filler under acidic conditions over 7 days could be maintained at the level required to hinder *S. mutans* and multi-species biofilm formation in vitro [35]. However, F^- release from both the GIC-containing BioUnion filler and Fuji VII gradually decreased over 7 days, and its concentrations, although higher under acidic conditions, were below the level required to inhibit *S. mutans* and multi-species biofilm formation in vitro. Furthermore, they indicated that the GIC used in this study could recharge the Zn^{2+} and F^- in the BioUnion filler. Although there were no significant differences in the results obtained in this study, considering that Caredyne ZIF-C is expected to have a sustained anti-biofilm effect due to Zn^{2+} in addition to F- and that its fall-out rate tended to be lower than that of Fuji VII, Caredyne ZIF-C might be more suitable than Fuji VII as a tooth-coating material for initial active root caries. We look forward to the results from future large-scale clinical studies.

This study has some limitations, including its small sample size. Taking the results of this study into consideration, the calculated sample size should be around 140 subjects per group. Future research should include large multi-center prospective studies. Another limitation was the fact that changes in cement-coated tooth surfaces were difficult to evaluate unless the tooth-coating materials were removed. Therefore, the root caries preventive rate or caries arrest rate could not be evaluated, and the only parameter that could be evaluated regarding caries progression was the failure rate, defined as the need for restoration due to caries progression. There were no significant differences in failure rates among the groups, suggesting that root caries stabilization among the materials may be comparable. However, one or two teeth in each group needed restoration, and measuring dentin hardness may have allowed for a more detailed evaluation of the differences among the materials. Therefore, we are considering an evaluation of the possibility of removing the cement without damaging the caries lesion. Additionally, it is desirable to evaluate hardness in future research.

Based on the results of this pilot study, to verify the potential of GICs as coating materials against initial active root caries, it is necessary to improve the evaluation method for lesion surface hardness. Additionally, it is necessary to reevaluate the timing of evaluation and determine the appropriate control for plaque attachment, as stated earlier. Further research on this aspect is warranted.

5. Conclusions

Although no significant differences were noted in the failure rate and plaque attachment rate among GICs coating and fluoride application, several areas for improvement in the methods were noted for future research. Thus, this pilot study is the first step of a clinical study using GICs as the tooth-coating materials for initial active root caries, and it forms the foundation of the main study. Although fluoride application is the gold standard in the field of root caries management, this pilot study may offer a new direction in the management of initial active root caries, in which additional effects by coating can be expected in addition to the anti-carious effects of GICs. Caredyne ZIF-C can especially be expected to have anti-biofilm and anti-demineralization effects not only due to F^- but also due to Zn^{2+}. Although there was no significant difference, the fall-out rate tended to be lower than that of Fuji VII; therefore, it might be more desirable as a tooth-coating material for the secondary prevention of root caries. As the next steps in research, we are planning a study to assess the possibility of removing cement materials without damaging the tooth surface to evaluate the latter's hardness. Further, we are planning to conduct a larger clinical trial that employs the contemplated approach for quantifying tooth hardness, along with enhanced methodologies for assessing the rate of plaque attachment.

Supplementary Materials: The following supporting information can be downloaded at https://www.mdpi.com/article/10.3390/medicina60010150/s1: Table S1: Characteristics of teeth in which material fall-out was observed.

Author Contributions: Conceptualization, M.H., Y.N., H.Y. and Y.A.; methodology, M.H, Y.N. and H.Y.; formal analysis, H.K. and Y.A.; investigation, K.N. (Katsuaki Naito), K.N. (Kazuaki Niwano) and D.T.; data curation, Y.A.; writing—original draft preparation, Y.A.; writing—review and editing, M.H., Y.N. and H.Y.; supervision, M.H, Y.N. and H.Y.; project administration, M.H.; funding acquisition, Y.A. All authors have read and agreed to the published version of the manuscript.

Funding: This research was funded by JSPS KAKENHI (Grant Numbers JP20K09953 and JP23K09198).

Institutional Review Board Statement: This study was conducted in accordance with the Declaration of Helsinki and approved on 8 January 2019 by the Ethics Committees of the Osaka University Graduate School of Dentistry (H30-E40-3), Niigata University (2019-0007), and Tokushima University Hospital (3573-3). Trial registration: UMIN Clinical Trials Registry (UMIN-CTR), UMIN000035609. Registered on 22 January 2019.

Informed Consent Statement: Informed consent was obtained from all the subjects involved in this study.

Data Availability Statement: The data presented in this study are available upon reasonable request from the corresponding author. The data cannot be publicly accessed owing to disagreements among the study participants.

Acknowledgments: We thank Hijiri Masuda, Chiaki Oizumi, Makoto Hirohara, Yoko Ishihara, and Keisuke Ikushima of the GC Dental Industrial Corporation for providing Caredyne ZIF-C and Fuji VII.

Conflicts of Interest: The authors declare no conflicts of interest. The funders had no role in the design of the study, in the collection; analyses; or interpretation of the data, in the writing of the manuscript, or in the decision to publish the results.

References

1. Hariyani, N.; Setyowati, D.; Spencer, A.J.; Luzzi, L.; Do, L.G. Root caries incidence and increment in the population—A systematic review, meta-analysis and meta-regression of longitudinal studies. *J. Dent.* **2018**, *77*, 1–7. [CrossRef] [PubMed]
2. Chan, A.K.Y.; Tamrakar, M.; Jiang, C.M.; Lo, E.C.M.; Leung, K.C.M.; Chu, C.H. A systematic review on caries status of older adults. *Int. J. Environ. Res. Public Health* **2021**, *18*, 10662. [CrossRef] [PubMed]

3. Bignozzi, I.; Crea, A.; Capri, D.; Littarru, C.; Lajolo, C.; Tatakis, D.N. Root caries: A periodontal perspective. *J. Periodont. Res.* **2014**, *49*, 143–163. [CrossRef] [PubMed]
4. Momoi, Y.; Hayashi, M.; Fujitani, M.; Fukushima, M.; Imazato, S.; Kubo, S.; Nikaido, T.; Shimizu, A.; Unemori, M.; Yamaki, C. Clinical guidelines for treating caries in adults following a minimal intervention policy–evidence and consensus based report. *J. Dent.* **2012**, *40*, 95–105. [CrossRef]
5. Schwendicke, F.; Gostemeyer, G. Cost-effectiveness of root caries preventive treatments. *J. Dent.* **2017**, *56*, 58–64. [CrossRef]
6. Gluzman, R.; Katz, R.V.; Frey, B.J.; McGowan, R. Prevention of root caries: A literature review of primary and secondary preventive agents. *Spec. Care Dentist* **2013**, *33*, 133–140. [CrossRef]
7. Wierichs, R.J.; Meyer-Lueckel, H. Systematic review on noninvasive treatment of root caries lesions. *J. Dent. Res.* **2015**, *94*, 261–271. [CrossRef]
8. Urquhart, O.; Tampi, M.P.; Pilcher, L.; Slayton, R.L.; Araujo, M.W.B.; Fontana, M.; Guzmán-Armstrong, S.; Nascimento, M.M.; Nový, B.B.; Tinanoff, N.; et al. Nonrestorative treatments for caries: Systematic review and network meta-analysis. *J. Dent. Res.* **2019**, *98*, 14–26. [CrossRef]
9. Wicht, M.J.; Haak, R.; Lummert, D.; Noack, M.J. Treatment of root caries lesions with chlorhexidine-containing varnishes and dentin sealants. *Am. J. Dent.* **2003**, *16*, 25A–30A.
10. Baysan, A.; Lynch, E. Clinical reversal of root caries using ozone: 6-month results. *Am. J. Dent.* **2007**, *20*, 203–208.
11. Grogono, A.L.; Mayo, J.A. Prevention of root caries with dentin adhesives. *Am. J. Dent.* **1994**, *7*, 89–90. [PubMed]
12. Swift, E.J.; Hammel, S.A.; Perdigao, J.; Wefel, J.S. Prevention of root surface caries using a dental adhesive. *J. Am. Dent. Assoc.* **1994**, *125*, 571–576. [CrossRef] [PubMed]
13. Cai, J.; Palamara, J.; Manton, D.J.; Burrow, M.F. Status and progress of treatment methods for root caries in the last decade: A literature review. *Aust. Dent. J.* **2018**, *63*, 34–54. [CrossRef] [PubMed]
14. Hayes, M.; Brady, P.; Burke, F.M.; Allen, P.F. Failure rates of class V restorations in the management of root caries in adults—A systematic review. *Gerodontology* **2016**, *33*, 299–307. [CrossRef] [PubMed]
15. Wiegand, A.; Buchalla, W.; Attin, T. Review on fluoride-releasing restorative materials--fluoride release and uptake characteristics, antibacterial activity and influence on caries formation. *Dent. Mater.* **2007**, *23*, 343–362. [CrossRef]
16. Burgess, J.O.; Gallo, J.R. Treating root-surface caries. *Dent. Clin. North Am.* **2002**, *46*, 385–404. [CrossRef]
17. Neves, A.B.; Bergstrom, T.G.; Fonseca-Goncalves, A.; Dos Santos, T.M.P.; Lopes, R.T.; de Almeida Neves, A. Mineral density changes in bovine carious dentin after treatment with bioactive dental cements: A comparative micro-CT study. *Clin. Oral Investig.* **2019**, *23*, 1865–1870. [CrossRef]
18. Trairatvorakul, C.; Itsaraviriyakul, S.; Wiboonchan, W. Effect of glass-ionomer cement on the progression of proximal caries. *J. Dent. Res.* **2011**, *90*, 99–103. [CrossRef]
19. Munoz-Sandoval, C.; Gambetta-Tessini, K.; Giacaman, R.A. Microcavitated (ICDAS 3) carious lesion arrest with resin or glass ionomer sealants in first permanent molars: A randomized controlled trial. *J. Dent.* **2019**, *88*, 103163. [CrossRef]
20. Imazato, S.; Kohno, T.; Tsuboi, R.; Thongthai, P.; Xu, H.H.; Kitagawa, H. Cutting-edge filler technologies to release bio-active components for restorative and preventive dentistry. *Dent. Mater. J.* **2020**, *39*, 69–79. [CrossRef]
21. Hasegawa, T.; Takenaka, S.; Ohsumi, T.; Ida, T.; Ohshima, H.; Terao, Y.; Naksagoon, T.; Maeda, T.; Noiri, Y. Effect of a novel glass ionomer cement containing fluoro-zinc-silicate fillers on biofilm formation and dentin ion incorporation. *Clin. Oral Investig.* **2020**, *24*, 963–970. [CrossRef] [PubMed]
22. Liu, Y.; Kohno, T.; Tsuboi, R.; Kitagawa, H.; Imazato, S. Acidity-induced release of zinc ion from BioUnion™ filler and its inhibitory effects against Streptococcus mutans. *Dent. Mater. J.* **2020**, *39*, 547–553. [CrossRef] [PubMed]
23. Saad, A.; Nikaido, T.; Abdou, A.; Matin, K.; Burrow, M.F.; Tagami, J. Inhibitory effect of zinc-containing desensitizer on bacterial biofilm formation and root dentin demineralization. *Dent. Mater. J.* **2019**, *38*, 940–946. [CrossRef] [PubMed]
24. Takatsuka, T.; Tanaka, K.; Iijima, Y. Inhibition of dentine demineralization by zinc oxide: In vitro and in situ studies. *Dent. Mater.* **2005**, *21*, 1170–1177. [CrossRef]
25. Toledano, M.; Yamauti, M.; Osorio, E.; Osorio, R. Zinc-inhibited MMP-mediated collagen degradation after different dentine demineralization procedures. *Caries Res.* **2012**, *46*, 201–217. [CrossRef]
26. Takahashi, K.; Shimada, Y.; Tagami, J.; Yoshiyama, M. The effects of root demineralization inhibition by a glass ionomer cement containing zinc glass. *Jpn. J. Conserv. Dent.* **2019**, *62*, 190–198.
27. He, G.; Pearce, E.I.; Sissons, C.H. Inhibitory effect of $ZnCl_2$ on glycolysis in human oral microbes. *Arch. Oral Biol.* **2002**, *47*, 117–129. [CrossRef] [PubMed]
28. Pitts, N. "ICDAS"—An international system for caries detection and assessment being developed to facilitate caries epidemiology, research and appropriate clinical management. *Community Dent. Health.* **2004**, *21*, 193–198.
29. Yoshida, A.; Suzuki, N.; Nakano, Y.; Kawada, M.; Oho, T.; Koga, T. Development of a 5′ nuclease-based real-time PCR assay for quantitative detection of cariogenic dental pathogens Streptococcus mutans and Streptococcus sobrinus. *J. Clin. Microbiol.* **2003**, *41*, 4438–4441. [CrossRef]
30. Hellyer, P.H.; Beighton, D.; Heath, M.R.; Lynch, E.J. Root caries in older people attending a general dental practice in East Sussex. *Br. Dent. J.* **1990**, *169*, 201–206. [CrossRef]
31. Momoi, Y.; Shimizu, A.; Hayashi, M.; Imazato, S.; Unemori, M.; Kitasako, Y.; Kubo, S.; Takahashi, R.; Nakashima, S.; Nikaido, T.; et al. Root caries management: Evidence and consensus based report. *Curr. Oral Health Rep.* **2016**, *3*, 117–123. [CrossRef]

32. Lancaster, G.A.; Dodd, S.; Williamson, P.R. Design and analysis of pilot studies: Recommendations for good practice. *J. Eval. Clin. Pract.* **2004**, *10*, 307–312. [CrossRef] [PubMed]
33. Nagasawa, Y.; Eda, Y.; Matsumoto, S.; Nakajima, H.; Hibino, Y. Bond strength of encapsulated Zn-containing glass ionomer cement to dentin. *Jpn. J. Conserv. Dent.* **2021**, *64*, 141–155.
34. Nishida, E.; Miyaji, H.; Shitomi, K.; Sugaya, T.; Akasaka, T. Evaluation of antibacterial and cytocompatible properties of multiple-ion releasing zinc-fluoride glass nanoparticles. *Dent. Mater. J.* **2021**, *40*, 157–164. [CrossRef]
35. Kohno, T.; Liu, Y.; Tsuboi, R.; Kitagawa, H.; Imazato, S. Evaluation of ion release and the recharge ability of glass-ionomer cement containing BioUnion filler using an in vitro saliva-drop setting assembly. *Dent. Mater.* **2021**, *37*, 882–893. [CrossRef]

Disclaimer/Publisher's Note: The statements, opinions and data contained in all publications are solely those of the individual author(s) and contributor(s) and not of MDPI and/or the editor(s). MDPI and/or the editor(s) disclaim responsibility for any injury to people or property resulting from any ideas, methods, instructions or products referred to in the content.

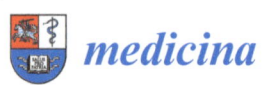

Article

Silver Diamine Fluoride Renaissance in Paediatric Dentistry: A 24-Month Retrospective and Cross-Sectional Analysis

Ruba Abdulrahim [1], Christian H. Splieth [1], Mhd Said Mourad [1,2], Annina Vielhauer [1], Manasi R. Khole [1] and Ruth M. Santamaría [1,*]

[1] Department of Preventive and Pediatric Dentistry, University of Greifswald, 17475 Greifswald, Germany; ruba.abdulrahim@stud.uni-greifswald.de (R.A.); splieth@uni-greifswald.de (C.H.S.); mhd.mourad@uni-greifswald.de (M.S.M.); annina.vielhauer@uni-greifswald.de (A.V.); manasi.khole1@uni-greifswald.de (M.R.K.)

[2] Department of Orthodontics, University of Greifswald, 17475 Greifswald, Germany

* Correspondence: ruth.santamaria@uni-greifswald.de; Tel.: +49-383-486-7167

Abstract: *Background and Objectives:* Silver diamine fluoride (SDF) has been incorporated into the treatment of dental caries in children, mainly in countries with high caries prevalence. In Europe, however, SDF started to gain popularity during the COVID-19 pandemic. This study aimed to investigate the efficacy of SDF and to evaluate dentists'/parents' acceptance of SDF use in paediatric patients treated in a German university setting. *Materials and Methods:* A retrospective analysis of all patients treated with SDF between 2017 and 2020 was carried out. Only teeth with no reported clinical/radiographic evidence of irreversible pulpal inflammation were included. The outcome measures were success, minor failures (caries progression, reversible pulpitis) and major failures (irreversible pulpitis, abscess). The treatment acceptance by dentists and the parents of SDF-treated children was cross-sectionally evaluated using questionnaires. Descriptive statistics and Kaplan–Meier survival analysis were performed. *Results:* A total of 93 patients (mean age 5.3 ± 2.9 years) with 455 treated teeth (418 primary/91.9%; 37 permanent/8.1%) were included and followed up for up to 24 months (19.9 ± 10.5 months). SDF was used for dental caries (98.2%) and hypersensitivity relief on MIH teeth (1.8%). Most teeth did not show any failure (total success 84.2%). A total of 5 teeth (1.1%) showed minor failures, and 67 teeth (14.7%) showed major failures ($p = 0.001$). Success/failure rates were not affected by patient compliance, gender, dentition, or operator ($p > 0.05$). In total, 30 questionnaires were collected from parents (mean age 36.8 ± 6.4 years). SDF was applied on anterior ($n = 2/6.7\%$), posterior ($n = 15/50\%$) and anterior/posterior teeth ($n = 13/43.3\%$). At the 1-week follow-up, 80% of parents noticed black teeth discoloration. Treatment satisfaction was higher for posterior (95.2%) than for anterior teeth (36.4%; $p < 0.001$). In the 27 responses from clinicians, SDF was generally considered a viable option in paediatric dentistry ($n = 23$; 85%). *Conclusions:* SDF was found to be effective and well-accepted by parents and dentists for caries inactivation in a paediatric dentistry German university setting.

Keywords: dental caries; silver diamine fluoride; treatment outcome; paediatric dentistry; parents

Citation: Abdulrahim, R.; Splieth, C.H.; Mourad, M.S.; Vielhauer, A.; Khole, M.R.; Santamaría, R.M. Silver Diamine Fluoride Renaissance in Paediatric Dentistry: A 24-Month Retrospective and Cross-Sectional Analysis. *Medicina* **2024**, *60*, 16. https://doi.org/10.3390/medicina60010016

Academic Editor: Gaetano Isola

Received: 19 October 2023
Revised: 8 December 2023
Accepted: 19 December 2023
Published: 21 December 2023

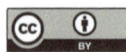

Copyright: © 2023 by the authors. Licensee MDPI, Basel, Switzerland. This article is an open access article distributed under the terms and conditions of the Creative Commons Attribution (CC BY) license (https://creativecommons.org/licenses/by/4.0/).

1. Introduction

Dental caries in children remain a global oral health issue to this day. Multiple risk factors have been associated with this issue, such as poor oral hygiene and dietary habits as well as altered oral bacterial flora. The increasing prevalence, especially in countries with low socio-economic status, present as a burden and challenge to its management. Hence, biological-based minimally invasive treatment strategies have been widely advocated in the recent literature [1]. First developed in the late 1960s, silver diamine fluoride (SDF) has been a research topic of interest, particularly in the last decade [2]. It has been thoroughly investigated and several systematic reviews have demonstrated its effectiveness in arresting caries in primary teeth, showing up to 91% success rates with biannual application [3–5]. This led the World Health Organisation to list it as an essential medicine for the treatment of carious lesions [6]. SDF has been largely researched in countries with high caries prevalence and regions with limited access to dental care [7–9].

The growing evidence on its effectiveness has led to its adoption worldwide including, but not limited to, in Australia, Brazil, Hong Kong, Japan, and the United States [10]. On the other hand, in Europe, treatment with SDF has been very limited due to the lack of national guidelines and its restricted off-label use. It has been proposed as an alternative option for young children presenting with high caries levels or low cooperation for invasive restorative therapy. In this regard, the European Organisation for Caries Research (ORCA), the European Federation of Conservative Dentistry (EFCD) as well as the German Association of Conservative Dentistry (DGZ) published, in a recent consensus statement, a recommendation of high-strength that SDF can be successfully used in the treatment of ECC [11]. SDF became further widespread during the COVID-19 pandemic, as it is considered as a non-invasive, non-aerosol-generating procedure [10,12].

Considering the lack of research on SDF use in Europe, this study aimed to investigate the clinical efficacy and acceptance by dentists and parents of paediatric patients treated with SDF application in Germany in a university dental setting.

2. Materials and Methods

2.1. Ethical Approval and Study Outline

Ethical approval was obtained from the Research Ethics Committee of the University of Greifswald under protocol number BB-142/20. This study comprised two different designs: a retrospective analysis and a cross-sectional questionnaire-based analysis.

2.2. Retrospective Analysis

Electronic records of all patients treated with SDF at the Preventive and Paediatric Dentistry Department in the University of Greifswald, Germany were retrospectively collected and followed up to evaluate the effectiveness of SDF treatment.

Study sample and inclusion and exclusion criteria

All patients, irrespective of age or health status, without baseline clinical or radiographic signs/symptoms of pulpal/periapical pathology, who were treated with SDF at the University of Greifswald Paediatric Department between January 2017 and February 2020, and who had attended at least one follow-up appointment (until February 2022), were included in the study. Patient records with insufficient documentation were excluded.

Clinical procedure

The SDF product used was Riva Star® (SDI Limited, Victoria 3153, Australia), which includes two bottles that are applied sequentially: bottle/step 1 corresponds to 38% SDF solution and bottle/step 2 contains potassium iodide (KI) solution (to lower the risk of black staining). The tooth is first cleaned, and debris removed. Soft tissues are protected using cotton rolls and petroleum jelly. SDF solution is then applied on the carious lesion using a micro brush after drying the tooth. The treatment was performed in a chairside setting by 8 dentists, 5 of whom were paediatric dental specialists and 3 were postgraduate paediatric dentistry (PD) students with at least 2 years of working experience, all following the department's standard protocol for caries management in children and trained in treating children with SDF.

Outcomes

Recorded data comprised demographics (age, gender, address, medical status) and clinical baseline findings (d_3mft/s-D_3MFT/S index, clinical diagnosis, severity level of carious lesions using ICDAS index, radiographic and pulpal status, etc.). Outcome measures were assessed according to the last follow-up session using criteria modified from Innes et al. (2006) (Table 1) [13]. Data collection was based on the documentation obtained from the dental records. Documentation following treatment at the Preventive and Paediatric Dentistry Department was completed in a thorough and standardised manner using pre-set text for each procedure with the possibility to add or change notes when needed. Only patients with the sufficient documentation necessary for the study were included. Similarly, data were collected and decoded by the main investigator (RA) and reviewed by at least one co-investigator each time in a standardised manner using a Microsoft Excel (2020) spreadsheet prepared for the purpose of this study with the above-mentioned variables.

Table 1. Assessment criteria for the outcome analysis of treated teeth considering the two indications for SDF use.

Success
Dental caries
• Caries arrested (hardness/softness; lesion feels hard on gentle probing; characteristic SDF discoloration/black staining reported) and no further treatment required. • Caries arrested and tooth restored. • No clinical signs or symptoms of irreversible pulpal pathology. • Tooth exfoliated without minor or major failure.
Dentin hypersensitivity (due to MIH)
• Reported reduced MIH hypersensitivity, tooth not restored. • Reported reduced MIH hypersensitivity, tooth then restored.
Minor Failure
Dental caries
• Caries progression (hardness/softness; soft/leathery lesion on gentle probing; partially achieved/no reported SDF discoloration/black staining). • Signs or symptoms of reversible pulpitis treated without requiring pulpotomy or extraction.
Dentin hypersensitivity (due to MIH)
• Hypersensitivity persisted and required other treatment without pulpotomy or extraction.
Major Failure
• Signs or symptoms of reversible pulpitis (no spontaneous pain) requiring pulpotomy. • Signs or symptoms of irreversible pulpitis (spontaneous/persistent pain) or dental abscess requiring pulpectomy or extraction.

2.3. Cross-Sectional Questionnaire-Based Analysis

Questionnaires were created to assess dentists' and parents' acceptance of SDF treatment in children. The created questionnaires were first pilot tested with two paediatric dentists and five parents to ensure that they were comprehensible and acceptable to the target groups. No major flaws in the design of the questionnaires were revealed and the participating parents did not report any difficulty in answering the questions. Minor changes regarding the questionnaire structure, language, and format were made.

Sample size calculation

For the dentists' questionnaire, all identified dentists using SDF at the University of Greifswald Paediatric Department were invited to participate in the study. However, for the parents' questionnaire, the sample size was calculated according to initial results of the retrospective analysis (see Section 3.1). By assuming that around 400 patients received SDF annually, the sample size was calculated with population size = 400, confidence level 95% and a margin of error 20%, which, in turn, resulted in at least 23 participants to be included. Adding loss of responses due to missing data in the questionnaires (about 30%), a total sample size of 30 parents was determined.

Study participants
Parents/caregivers

The main investigator (RA) screened regular clinic attendees for eligible patients and consecutively recruited 30 participants according to the inclusion criteria. Only parents whose children were to be treated with SDF and who fully completed the first and follow-up questionnaires were included.

After obtaining a signed informed consent form, two questionnaires were distributed to the parents before and after one week of SDF application. The first questionnaire included a 12-item fill-in and Likert-scale questions covering participants' demographics and assessing parents' perception of the SDF procedure performed in terms of child comfort and behaviour during application and treatment duration. Meanwhile, the follow-up questionnaire consisted of 14-item fill-in and Likert-scale questions. The primary survey question was whether dark staining on the treated teeth was noticed by the parents or not, and if noticed, their opinion about it. Possible responses ranged from "very acceptable" to "very unacceptable". The secondary questions further explored parents' opinion of 3 main aspects related to the treatment: aesthetics, pain/complaints and SDF as a treatment option of carious lesions.

Dental practitioners

The dentists surveyed included paediatric dental specialists and post-graduate PD students all treating children on a regular basis. The questionnaire included 4 fill-in items regarding dentists' experience and qualifications and 12 Likert-scale statements aimed at exploring dentists' acceptance and experience with SDF. Possible responses ranged from "totally agree" to "totally disagree". To explore acceptance, dentists were asked if they considered SDF a good treatment option for ECC or avoided it due to the associated black staining.

2.4. Statistical Analysis

Statistical analysis was carried out using SPSS (IBM Corp. Released 2017. IBM SPSS Statistics for Mac, Version 25.0. Armonk, NY, USA: IBM Corp.). Descriptive statistics were applied to describe patient characteristics and conditions of treated teeth. Chi-square statistics were used to test relationships between categorical variables. Survival analysis using the Mantel–Cox method and a Kaplan–Meier curve were used to report mean time until treatment failure as well as the Log-rank test. A Mann–Whitney U test was performed to test the differences in the acceptance of SDF treatment. The level of significance was set at 0.05.

3. Results

3.1. Patient Profiles and Characteristics

The dental records of 1202 patients were initially retrieved. The data were filtered and assessed according to the inclusion criteria. In total, 93 patients had sufficient documentation and attended at least one follow-up appointment. The demographic and clinical characteristics are presented in Table 2.

Table 2. Demographics and clinical characteristics of the study sample.

Characteristics (n = 93)		
Age, mean (SD)		5.3 years (2.9)
Gender, n (%)	Female	45 (48.4)
	Male	48 (51.6)
Caries experience, mean (SD)	$d_3$mft	6.3 (4.1)
	d_3t	4.9 (3.9)
	D_3MFT	2.5 (3.7)
	D_3T	1.6 (2.8)
Medical history, n (%)	Medically unfit	13 (14)
	Medically fit	80 (86)

SD = standard deviation; d = decay; m = missing; f = filled; t = teeth.

The patients' age ranged from 1 to 17 years (±5.3 years). A sum of 455 teeth were treated with an average of 4.9 teeth per patient. Most of the treated teeth were primary teeth (n = 418; 92%). Only 41 patients (44%) had a recent radiograph available within the last year, almost all (93%) showing carious lesions at the dentin level (ICDAS 4–6). A total of 52% of the patients had a very negative or negative cooperative level. Dental caries was the main reported diagnosis (98.2%), along with a few cases of hypersensitivity due to MIH (n = 8; 1.8%). Patients mean d_3mft/D_3MFT was 6.3/2.5. The patients were treated by a postgraduate paediatric dentistry student (46.2%) or by a paediatric dental specialist (53.8%). Regarding the side effects of SDF application, only a few cases of sensitivity (7.5%) were reported during the application of the product. Other than the black staining of the carious lesions (98%), no adverse effects were reported in this study.

3.2. Clinical Efficacy and Indication

After 2 years of SDF application (19.9; SD = 10.5 months), follow-up data were collected, and the outcome of the treatment was evaluated according to the success/failure criteria (Table 3). The SDF treatment showed an overall success rate of 84.2%. There were 5 teeth (1.1%) presenting with minor failures and 67 teeth (14.7%) with major failures (p = 0.001). Besides dental caries, SDF was also used in the treatment of MIH-associated hypersensitivity in permanent first molars. Out of the eight treated permanent first molars, five required further restorative treatment due to persisted hypersensitivity, and one was extracted under general anaesthesia. Excluding MIH, the success rate of treated teeth due to dental caries was 85.2% with around two-thirds (57.2%) of carious teeth arrested, but not restored. The other 42.8% of teeth were restored after lesion inactivation.

Table 3. Treatment outcome of SDF-treated teeth due to dental caries only.

Outcomes n (%)		Treatments Performed	n (%)
Success * 381 (85.2)	No restorative treatment performed 218 (57.2)	Further follow-ups **	218 (48.8)
	Further restorative treatment performed 163 (42.8)	SMART-Hall using PMC	79 (17.6)
		Filling (Composite/Compomer)	50 (11.2)
		SMART-Technique with GIC	22 (4.9)
		Anterior strip crowns	12 (2.7)
Minor Failure	Caries progression/Secondary caries 0 (0)		
Major Failure 66 (14.8)	Irreversible pulpitis/Abscess 66 (100)	Extraction	55 (12.3)
		Pulpotomy	11 (2.5)
Total			447

* Caries arrested; no signs/symptoms of irreversible pulpal pathology. ** Oral hygiene follow-ups involve bacterial plaque disclosing, tooth-brushing training, fluoride use, and application according to age, parental/patient active involvement, motivation, and reinforcement, etc. Glass Ionomer Cement (GIC): Silver Modified Atraumatic Restorative Treatment (SMART). SMART-Hall: after SDF application, teeth are restored using preformed metal crowns (PMC).

After SDF application, the mean survival time for primary and permanent teeth was 38.8 months (95% confidence interval 37.2 to 40.3) and 28.3 months (95% confidence interval 23.7 to 32.8), respectively (Figure 1). The log-rank test was run to compare the primary and permanent dentition in terms of time until failure. No significant difference between both groups was found (p = 0.19). The results of the study were not statistically significant when success/failure rates were compared according to patient compliance, gender, dentition, or medical condition ($p > 0.05$).

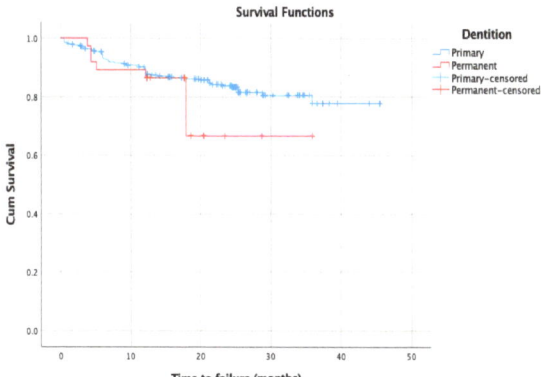

Figure 1. Kaplan–Meier survival curve showing survival time of SDF-treated teeth until failure.

3.3. Parents' Acceptance and Satisfaction

Initially, 42 responses were collected. In total, 30 participants fully completed the follow-up questionnaire and were included in the study. The participant parent was mainly the mother of the child ($n = 27$; 90%) with a mean age of 37 years (± 6.4 SD). SDF treatment was used on anterior teeth in 2 children (6.7%), posterior teeth in 15 children (50%), and both anterior and posterior in 13 children (43.3%). The parents had varying educational backgrounds from secondary school (5%) up to postgraduate studies (19%), with around 46% of parents having completed an apprenticeship, i.e., a vocational training programme. Among other reasons like regular check-up (27%) and pain (10%), the main reason behind the dental visit was dental caries in 63% of the participants.

At the first visit, there was an overall acceptance (70%) of the procedure in terms of child comfort. At the follow-up, 80% of the parents noticed dark staining on the treated teeth but around 71% assessed the treatment received as very acceptable or acceptable. However, satisfaction with treatment was higher for posterior teeth (95.2%) than for anterior teeth (36.4%; $p < 0.001$). When asked about the need for an aesthetic restoration, 43.3% responded with 'agree'. Around 93% responded with 'disagree' when asked if they regret receiving the treatment due to its discoloration and 97% chose 'agree' for using SDF to arrest caries. Overall, there was high acceptance of SDF treatment of caries among the participating parents (Figure 2).

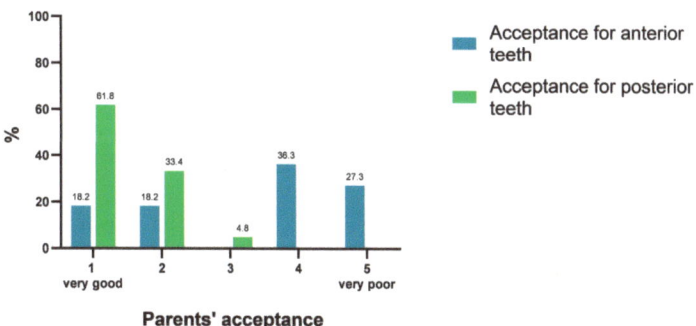

Figure 2. Parents' acceptance of dark staining associated with SDF treatment. Likert Scale (1–5) from very good to very poor acceptance of dark discoloration.

3.4. Dentists' Experience and Knowledge

In total, 27 responses were obtained. Among these, 56% ($n = 15$) were paediatric specialists, 11% ($n = 3$) dental practitioners, and 33% ($n = 9$) post-graduate students, all treating paediatric patients on a regular basis.

All participants in this study, expect one, confirmed their awareness of the SDF protocol. Around 60% (n = 16) of the respondents agreed that they confidently use SDF based on the researched evidence for its effectiveness. The importance of obtaining a consent form from the parents was also confirmed by all participants.

Most of the participants (n = 23; 85%) consider the use of SDF as a good treatment option for ECC, and 67% (n = 18) would prefer it over other treatment options for children with ECC, as well as for the treatment of carious lesions in anxious/low cooperative children (n = 22; 81%). All participants, except one (96%) who "somewhat disagrees", believe that SDF can be considered as an interim procedure to arrest carious lesions and win time until a restorative therapy can be delivered or until the child can be treated under general anaesthesia. Table 4 shows a summary of the main findings obtained from the questionnaire.

Table 4. Dentists' opinions of SDF treatment.

Questionnaire Item		n (%)
Find SDF a good alternative to the treatment of early childhood caries.	Agree	20 (74.1%)
	Somewhat agree	3 (11.1%)
	Neither	3 (11.1%)
	Somewhat disagree	1 (3.7%)
	Disagree	0 (0%)
Prefer SDF over other options for the treatment early childhood caries.	Agree	9 (33.3%)
	Somewhat agree	9 (33.3%)
	Neither	8 (29.6%)
	Somewhat disagree	1 (3.7%)
	Disagree	0 (0%)
Use SDF treatment for anxious children with caries.	Agree	10 (37%)
	Somewhat agree	12 (44.4%)
	Neither	3 (11.1%)
	Somewhat disagree	0 (0%)
	Disagree	2 (7.4%)
Consider SDF before restorative therapy or general anesthesia.	Agree	21 (77.8%)
	Somewhat agree	5 (18.5%)
	Neither	0 (0%)
	Somewhat disagree	1 (3.7%)
	Disagree	0 (0%)
Confidently use SDF based on the researched evidence for its effectiveness.	Agree	16 (59.3%)
	Somewhat agree	9 (33.3%)
	Neither	2 (7.4%)
	Somewhat disagree	0 (0%)
	Disagree	0 (0%)
Had an experience with parents rejecting SDF treatment due to aesthetics.	Agree	1 (3.7%)
	Somewhat agree	9 (33.3%)
	Neither	6 (22.2%)
	Somewhat disagree	9 (33.3%)
	Disagree	2 (7.4%)

4. Discussion

This study explored the use of SDF in terms of clinical efficacy (2-year follow-up) and acceptance by the dentists and parents of paediatric patients treated in Germany in a specialised university dental setting. SDF was primarily used to arrest active carious lesions in young patients (mean age = 5.3 years) presenting with high caries risk and experience ($d_3$mft/D_3MFT = 6.3/2.5) and low cooperation levels.

Regarding the caries experience of treated patients ($d_3$mft/D_3MFT of 6.3/2.5), these figures are particularly high in comparison to average values for children in primary and permanent dentition in Germany. For 3-year-olds, a weighted mean $d_3$mft value of 0.48 has been reported [14]. However, in the present study, this group presented almost 13 times higher d_3mft levels than the average value for the whole population. In addition, for the whole sample the "d_3/D_3" component of the d_3mft/D_3MFT index corresponded to 78% in primary teeth and 65% in permanent teeth of the whole caries experience. Considering the high treatment need of the whole sample, as well as the limited ability to cooperate with dental procedures at a young age, without SDF, the only likely treatment option would have been treatment under dental general anaesthesia (DGA). Although the clinical success of dental procedures under DGA is considered very high in the medium-term, this procedure increases the health risk for young patients as well as the economic burden for public health systems [15–17].

The selected caries management modality in this study followed recent guidelines and evidence-based recommendations on the use of non/minimally invasive treatment modalities like SDF [18,19]. In total, 455 teeth were treated, most of which were primary teeth (92%). An overall success rate of 84.2% of SDF-treated teeth after 2-year follow-up was observed. Excluding MIH teeth, the success rate of treated teeth increases to 85.2%. Several systematic reviews and an umbrella review have reported caries arrest rates ranging from 51% to 91% in primary teeth [20–23]. The studies included assessed the effectiveness of SDF in arresting carious lesions in children in comparison to a placebo, fluoride varnish, or the use of atraumatic restorative treatment, including anterior and posterior teeth, annual or biannual application and with varying concentrations of SDF. This explains the wide range reported according to each study and its setting. However, all systematic reviews agree that there is strong evidence for the efficacy of SDF in arresting carious lesions in children [24]. Similarly, the present study reported that 57.2% of the successfully SDF-treated carious teeth did not require any further treatment/restoration. The rest (42.8%) were further restored at subsequent visits mostly with GIC (SMART-Technique) or the Hall technique (SMART-Hall).

On the other hand, carious teeth categorised under failure were teeth that developed pathological signs/symptoms of irreversible pulp deterioration. Many of these teeth had to be treated with pulpotomy/extraction under DGA. The mean time after SDF application until DGA treatment was almost 1 year (10.7 months). So, even in these cases, SDF may be considered beneficial to buy time until an appointment for DGA could be arranged or to reduce the implied risks of DGA at young ages [17].

In this study, SDF was mainly used for the treatment of carious lesions; however, attempts to reduce dental hypersensitivity using SDF were also seen in a few cases of MIH. Since SDF is a dentin-desensitizing agent, its use in reducing dentin hypersensitivity associated with MIH is not novel [25]. The number of MIH-treated teeth in this study was small ($n = 8$) and most teeth required further restorative treatment to reduce hypersensitivity. In addition, due to the per se limitations of retrospective analyses, the severity of hypersensitivity and the degree of MIH could not be accurately reported in this study. It is therefore difficult to draw conclusions on the effectiveness of SDF in MIH-diagnosed teeth. However, one clinical trial has recently reported significant reductions in hypersensitivity following the application of SDF and SMART sealants on MIH teeth for up to one year [26].

Other than the dark staining of the carious lesions, no adverse effects were reported. In seven patients (7.5%), sensitivity upon application of the SDF solution was reported. Most of these patients were under 5 years of age and with a very negative or negative level of cooperation. This could explain the difficulty faced by the child receiving the treatment and perceiving it negatively. While SDF is biocompatible and safe to use [21], its direct application to vital pulp has been shown to cause pulpal necrosis [27]. Therefore, correct diagnosis is imperative prior to treatment with SDF in deep carious lesions.

A high response rate of 93% was obtained from the questionnaire distributed to the dentists who treated the patients in this study. Most participants considered SDF a viable treatment option for ECC, especially for young children presenting with dental anxiety and low compliance, since it is a simple procedure. Dental professionals in the UK have also reported similar views [28]. Also, almost all participants used SDF to buy time prior to restorative therapy or treatment under DGA. This opinion was also reported in a survey of paediatric dentists in the US [29]. Similar minimally invasive procedures for the treatment of caries in children, such as the Hall technique using preformed metal crowns and non-restorative caries control, were also found to be easy procedures for dentists and favoured by the children [30].

However, the dark staining side effect associated with SDF was reported by many practitioners as the main barrier to its use [28,31–33]. In this study, few dentists reported parents rejecting this treatment option due to aesthetic concerns. It was, therefore, crucial to explore parents' acceptance and satisfaction with SDF, since this product has been recently introduced and is not the most common treatment modality in Germany. Parents of treated children were surveyed prior to and after the application of SDF. Overall, parents showed a high acceptance of the procedure in terms of treatment time and child comfort and the majority assessed the treatment received as satisfactory with higher acceptance rates for posterior than for anterior teeth. A similar pattern was found in other studies that interviewed parents in the U.S. regarding their opinion of the discoloration following treatment with SDF [34,35], whereas a study from Saudi Arabia showed high disapproval rates, although the parents were interviewed and presented with photos and scenarios without the actual use of SDF [36]. It is important to note that the perception of aesthetics and beauty is subjective and influenced by several factors such as age, level of education and culture [37]. Child-related factors, such as the location of the tooth and cooperation level of the child, also play a role. One study reported high disapproval rates; however, when more advanced behavioural techniques such as DGA were avoided by treatment with SDF, the acceptance rates increased [38].

The results reported in this study should be interpreted alongside its limitations. The effectiveness of SDF treatment was evaluated by performing a retrospective analysis. While comparing results from a retrospective study to those of a clinical trial cannot be considered completely valid, the findings from this study represent long-term outcomes and the prognosis of the treated teeth after SDF application. An advantage of such a study is that the patients recruited have been regularly treated and the results are then assessed without pressure on practitioners being aware of participating in a clinical study. In addition, the analysis was carried out under the strict evaluation of the treated teeth using pre-set criteria determining the levels of success, minor or major failures. The surveying of dental professionals included participants employed or part of a post-graduate program at a university paediatric dentistry department; this may pose a concern as the findings cannot be generalised.

Lastly, future efforts should aim to incorporate different remineralising agents in addition to fluorides. A proactive action could be necessary to reduce the incidence of caries in children using products, such as substances based on biomimetic hydroxyapatite, that are showing similar potential in remineralisation [39]. Also, further research is needed to develop a clear treatment plan following SDF treatment. This includes longitudinal studies evaluating the success rates and longevity of direct restorative treatment after SDF application, such as GIC sealants and preformed metal crowns or the further inactivation of caries with multiple SDF applications.

5. Conclusions

To the best of our knowledge, this is the first time the use of SDF has been assessed in Germany. The findings of this study give an overview of the treatment of SDF in children and its acceptance by parents and dental practitioners. SDF was found to be effective in treating young children with high caries risk in the long-term, which was perceived as acceptable by dental practitioners and parents equally. We can, therefore, conclude that, with proper diagnosis and sufficient awareness of dentists and parents, SDF can be particularly beneficial for at-risk patients whose treatment could otherwise be very challenging.

Author Contributions: Conceptualisation, R.A., C.H.S. and R.M.S.; Investigation, R.A. and R.M.S.; Methodology, R.A., C.H.S. and R.M.S.; Resources, R.A., M.S.M. and A.V.; Supervision, R.M.S.; Writing—original draft, R.A.; Writing—review and editing, R.A., C.H.S., M.S.M., M.R.K. and R.M.S. All authors have read and agreed to the published version of the manuscript.

Funding: This research received no external funding.

Institutional Review Board Statement: The study was conducted in accordance with the Declaration of Helsinki and approved by the Ethics Committee of Greifswald University (protocol number BB-142/20 20.08.2020, approval date 20 August 2020).

Informed Consent Statement: Informed consent was obtained from all subjects involved in the study.

Data Availability Statement: The data are contained within the article. Further inquiries can be directed to the corresponding author.

Acknowledgments: The authors thank the parents and dentists who participated in this study.

Conflicts of Interest: The authors declare that they have no conflicts of interest.

References

1. Butera, A.; Maiorani, C.; Morandini, A.; Simonini, M.; Morittu, S.; Trombini, J.; Scribante, A. Evaluation of Children Caries Risk Factors: A Narrative Review of Nutritional Aspects, Oral Hygiene Habits, and Bacterial Alterations. *Children* **2022**, *9*, 262. [CrossRef] [PubMed]
2. Qasim, S.S.B.; Ali, D.; Khan, A.S.; Rehman, S.U.; Iqbal, A.; Baskaradoss, J.K. Evidence-Based Bibliometric Analysis of Research on Silver Diamine Fluoride Use in Dentistry. *BioMed Res. Int.* **2021**, *2021*, 9917408. [CrossRef] [PubMed]
3. Schmoeckel, J.; Gorseta, K.; Splieth, C.H.; Juric, H. How to Intervene in the Caries Process: Early Childhood Caries—A Systematic Review. *Caries Res.* **2020**, *54*, 102–112. [CrossRef] [PubMed]
4. BaniHani, A.; Santamaría, R.M.; Hu, S.; Maden, M.; Albadri, S. Minimal intervention dentistry for managing carious lesions into dentine in primary teeth: An umbrella review. *Eur. Arch. Paediatr. Dent.* **2022**, *23*, 667–693. [CrossRef] [PubMed]
5. Santamaría, R.M.; Abudrya, M.H.; Gül, G.; Mourad, M.S.; Gomez, G.F.; Zandona, A.G.F. How to Intervene in the Caries Process: Dentin Caries in Primary Teeth. *Caries Res.* **2020**, *54*, 306–323. [CrossRef]
6. World Health Organization. *WHO Model List of Essential Medicines-22nd List, 2021*; Technical Document; World Health Organization: Geneva, Switzerland, 2021.
7. Chu, C.; Lo, E.; Lin, H. Effectiveness of silver diamine fluoride and sodium fluoride varnish in arresting dentin caries in Chinese pre-school children. *J. Dent. Res.* **2002**, *81*, 767–770. [CrossRef]
8. dos Santos, V.E.; de Vasconcelos, F.M.; Ribeiro, A.G.; Rosenblatt, A. Paradigm shift in the effective treatment of caries in schoolchildren at risk. *Int. Dent. J.* **2012**, *62*, 47–51. [CrossRef]
9. Nguyen, Y.H.T.; Ueno, M.; Zaitsu, T.; Nguyen, T.; Kawaguchi, Y. Caries Arresting Effect of Silver Diamine Fluoride in Vietnamese Preschool Children. *Int. J. Clin. Prev. Dent.* **2017**, *13*, 147–154. [CrossRef]
10. Gao, S.S.; Amarquaye, G.; Arrow, P.; Bansal, K.; Bedi, R.; Campus, G.; Chen, K.J.; Chibinski, A.C.R.; Chinzorig, T.; Crystal, Y.O.; et al. Global Oral Health Policies and Guidelines: Using Silver Diamine Fluoride for Caries Control. *Front. Oral Heal.* **2021**, *2*, 685557. [CrossRef]
11. Splieth, C.H.; Banerjee, A.; Bottenberg, P.; Breschi, L.; Campus, G.; Ekstrand, K.R.; Giacaman, R.A.; Haak, R.; Hannig, M.; Hickel, R.; et al. How to Intervene in the Caries Process in Children: A Joint ORCA and EFCD Expert Delphi Consensus Statement. *Caries Res.* **2020**, *54*, 297–305. [CrossRef]
12. Al Masri, A.; Abudrya Mohamed, H.; Splieth, C.H.; Schmoeckel, J.; Mourad, M.S.; Santamaría, R.M. How did the COVID-19 pandemic lockdown affect dental emergency care in children? Retrospective study in a specialized pedodontic center. *Quintessence Int.* **2021**, *52*, 788–796. [CrossRef] [PubMed]
13. Innes, N.P.T.; Stirrups, D.R.; Evans, D.J.P.; Hall, N.; Leggate, M. A novel technique using preformed metal crowns for managing carious primary molars in general practice—A retrospective analysis. *Br. Dent. J.* **2006**, *200*, 451–454. [CrossRef] [PubMed]
14. Basner, R.; Santamaria, R.M.; Schmoeckel, J.; Schüler, E.; Splieth, C.H. *Epidemiologische Begleituntersuchungen zur Gruppenprophylaxe 2016*; DAJ-Deutsche Arbeitsgemeinschaft Für Jugendzahnpflege e. V: Bonn, Germany, 2018.
15. Al-Eheideb, A.A.; Herman, N.G. Outcomes of dental procedures performed on children under general anesthesia. *J. Clin. Pediatr. Dent.* **2003**, *27*, 181–183. [CrossRef] [PubMed]
16. Spera, A.L.; Saxen, M.A.; Yepes, J.F.; Jones, J.E.; Sanders, B.J. Office-Based Anesthesia: Safety and Outcomes in Pediatric Dental Patients. *Anesth. Prog.* **2017**, *64*, 144–152. [CrossRef]
17. FDA Drug Safety Communication: FDA Review Results in New Warnings about Using General Anesthetics and Sedation Drugs in Young Children and Pregnant Women. 2016. Available online: https://www.fda.gov/drugs/drug-safety-and-availability/fda-drug-safety-communication-fda-review-results-new-warnings-about-using-general-anesthetics-and (accessed on 11 September 2023).

18. Phantumvanit, P.; Makino, Y.; Ogawa, H.; Rugg-Gunn, A.; Moynihan, P.; Petersen, P.E.; Evans, W.; Feldens, C.A.; Lo, E.; Khoshnevisan, M.H.; et al. WHO Global Consultation on Public Health Intervention against Early Childhood Caries. *Community Dent. Oral Epidemiol.* **2018**, *46*, 280–287. [CrossRef]
19. Crystal, Y.O.; Marghalani, A.A.; Ureles, S.D.; Wright, J.T.; Sulyanto, R.; Divaris, K.; Fontana, M.; Graham, L. Use of silver diamine fluoride for dental caries management in children and adolescents, including those with special health care needs. *Pediatr. Dent.* **2017**, *39*, E135–E145. [CrossRef]
20. Zaffarano, L.; Salerno, C.; Campus, G.; Cirio, S.; Balian, A.; Karanxha, L.; Cagetti, M.G. Silver Diamine Fluoride (SDF) Efficacy in Arresting Cavitated Caries Lesions in Primary Molars: A Systematic Review and Metanalysis. *Int. J. Environ. Res. Public. Health* **2022**, *19*, 12917. [CrossRef]
21. Seifo, N.; Cassie, H.; Radford, J.R.; Innes, N.P.T. Silver diamine fluoride for managing carious lesions: An umbrella review. *BMC Oral. Health* **2019**, *19*, 145. [CrossRef]
22. Chibinski, A.C.; Wambier, L.M.; Feltrin, J.; Loguercio, A.D.; Wambier, D.S.; Reis, A. Silver Diamine Fluoride Has Efficacy in Controlling Caries Progression in Primary Teeth: A Systematic Review and Meta-Analysis. *Caries Res.* **2017**, *51*, 527–541. [CrossRef]
23. Gao, S.; Zhao, I.; Hiraishi, N.; Duangthip, D.; Mei, M.; Lo, E.; Chu, C. Clinical trials of silver diamine fluoride in arresting caries among children: A systematic review. *JDR Clin. Transl. Res.* **2016**, *1*, 201–210. [CrossRef]
24. Crystal, Y.O.; Niederman, R. Evidence-Based Dentistry Update on Silver Diamine Fluoride. *Dent. Clin. N. Am.* **2019**, *63*, 45–68. [CrossRef] [PubMed]
25. Seifo, N.; Robertson, M.; MacLean, J.; Blain, K.; Grosse, S.; Milne, R.; Seeballuck, C.; Innes, N. The use of silver diamine fluoride (SDF) in dental practice. *Br. Dent. J.* **2020**, *228*, 75–81. [CrossRef] [PubMed]
26. Ballikaya, E.; Ünverdi, G.E.; Cehreli, Z.C. Management of initial carious lesions of hypomineralized molars (MIH) with silver diamine fluoride or silver-modified atraumatic restorative treatment (SMART): 1-year results of a prospective, randomized clinical trial. *Clin. Oral Investig.* **2022**, *26*, 2197–2205. [CrossRef] [PubMed]
27. Zaeneldin, A.; Yu, O.Y.; Chu, C.-H. Effect of silver diamine fluoride on vital dental pulp: A systematic review. *J. Dent.* **2022**, *119*, 104066. [CrossRef] [PubMed]
28. Seifo, N.; Cassie, H.; Radford, J.; Innes, N. "It's really no more difficult than putting on fluoride varnish": A qualitative exploration of dental professionals' views of silver diamine fluoride for the management of carious lesions in children. *BMC Oral. Health* **2020**, *20*, 257. [CrossRef]
29. Antonioni, M.B.; Fontana, M.; Salzmann, L.B.; Inglehart, M.R. Pediatric Dentists' Silver Diamine Fluoride Education, Knowledge, Attitudes, and Professional Behavior: A National Survey. *J. Dent. Educ.* **2019**, *83*, 173–182. [CrossRef]
30. Santamaria, R.M.; Innes, N.P.; Machiulskiene, V.; Evans, D.J.; Alkilzy, M.; Splieth, C.H. Acceptability of different caries management methods for primary molars in a RCT. *Int. J. Paediatr. Dent.* **2015**, *25*, 9–17. [CrossRef]
31. Alajlan, G.; Alshaikh, H.; Alshamrani, L.; Alanezi, M.; Alarfaj, S.; AlSwayyed, T. Knowledge on and attitude toward silver diamine fluoride among Saudi dental practitioners in Riyadh public hospitals. *Clin. Cosmet. Investig. Dent.* **2020**, *12*, 399–407. [CrossRef]
32. Vollú, A.L.; Moreira, J.P.d.L.; Luiz, R.R.; Barja-Fidalgo, F.; Fonseca-Gonçalves, A. Survey of knowledge, attitudes and practices of brazilian dentists regarding silver diamine fluoride. *Pesqui. Bras. Odontopediatria Clin. Integr.* **2019**, *20*, 1–7. [CrossRef]
33. Magno, M.B.; da Silva, L.P.; Ferreira, D.M.; Barja-Fidalgo, F.; Fonseca-Gonçalves, A. Aesthetic perception, acceptability and satisfaction in the treatment of caries lesions with silver diamine fluoride: A scoping review. *Int. J. Paediatr. Dent.* **2019**, *29*, 257–266. [CrossRef]
34. Clemens, J.; Gold, J.; Chaffin, J. Effect and acceptance of silver diamine fluoride treatment on dental caries in primary teeth. *J. Public Health Dent.* **2018**, *78*, 63–68. [CrossRef] [PubMed]
35. Cernigliaro, D.; Kumar, A.; Northridge, M.E.; Wu, Y.; Troxel, A.B.; Cunha-Cruz, J.; Balzer, J.; Okuji, D.M. Caregiver satisfaction with interim silver diamine fluoride applications for their children with caries prior to operating room treatment or sedation. *J. Public Health Dent.* **2019**, *79*, 286–291. [CrossRef] [PubMed]
36. Alshammari, A.F.; Almuqrin, A.A.; Aldakhil, A.M.; Alshammari, B.H.; Lopez, J.N.J. Parental perceptions and acceptance of silver diamine fluoride treatment in Kingdom of Saudi Arabia. *Int. J. Health Sci.* **2019**, *13*, 25–29.
37. Vallittu, P.K.; Vallittu, A.S.J.; Lassila, V.P. Dental aesthetics—A survey of attitudes in different groups of patients. *J. Dent.* **1996**, *24*, 335–338. [CrossRef]
38. Crystal, Y.O.; Janal, M.N.; Hamilton, D.S.; Niederman, R. Parental perceptions and acceptance of silver diamine fluoride staining. *J. Am. Dent. Assoc.* **2017**, *148*, 510–518.e4. [CrossRef]
39. Butera, A.; Gallo, S.; Pascadopoli, M.; Montasser, M.A.; El Latief, M.H.A.; Modica, G.G.; Scribante, A. Home Oral Care with Biomimetic Hydroxyapatite vs. Conventional Fluoridated Toothpaste for the Remineralization and Desensitizing of White Spot Lesions: Randomized Clinical Trial. *Int. J. Environ. Res. Public Health* **2022**, *19*, 8676. [CrossRef]

Disclaimer/Publisher's Note: The statements, opinions and data contained in all publications are solely those of the individual author(s) and contributor(s) and not of MDPI and/or the editor(s). MDPI and/or the editor(s) disclaim responsibility for any injury to people or property resulting from any ideas, methods, instructions or products referred to in the content.

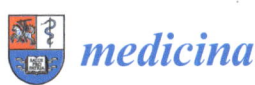

Article

Efficacy of Different Fluoride Therapies on Hypersensitive Carious Lesions in Primary Teeth

Mohamed Abudrya [1], Christian H. Splieth [1], Mhd Said Mourad [1,2] and Ruth M. Santamaría [1,*]

1. Department of Preventive and Pediatric Dentistry, University Medicine of Greifswald, 17475 Greifswald, Germany; mohamed.abudrya@stud.uni-greifswald.de (M.A.); splieth@uni-greifswald.de (C.H.S.); mhd.mourad@uni-greifswald.de (M.S.M.)
2. Department of Orthodontics, University Medicine of Greifswald, 17475 Greifswald, Germany
* Correspondence: ruth.santamaria@uni-greifswald.de; Tel.: +49-3834867167

Citation: Abudrya, M.; Splieth, C.H.; Mourad, M.S.; Santamaría, R.M. Efficacy of Different Fluoride Therapies on Hypersensitive Carious Lesions in Primary Teeth. *Medicina* **2023**, *59*, 2042. https://doi.org/10.3390/medicina59112042

Academic Editor: Bruno Chrcanovic

Received: 25 September 2023
Revised: 6 November 2023
Accepted: 7 November 2023
Published: 20 November 2023

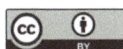

Copyright: © 2023 by the authors. Licensee MDPI, Basel, Switzerland. This article is an open access article distributed under the terms and conditions of the Creative Commons Attribution (CC BY) license (https://creativecommons.org/licenses/by/4.0/).

Abstract: *Background and Objectives:* This prospective, comparative, double-cohort study aimed to compare the efficacy of silver diamine fluoride and potassium iodide (38% SDF+KI; Riva Star®) with sodium fluoride varnish (5% NaF; Duraphat®) in hypersensitive carious lesions in primary teeth to evaluate caries arrest and hypersensitivity relief. *Materials and Methods:* This study included thirty 2–5-year-olds (mean age = 3.67 ± 1.06 years; 16 males and 14 females) who required a desensitizing treatment for hypersensitive carious defects with visible dentin. A total of 15 of the participants were consecutively allocated to treatment with 5% NaF, and they were further compared to an equal number of participants treated with 38% SDF+KI solutions (n = 15). The treatments were performed following clinical evaluation of caries activity using the International Caries Classification and Management System (ICCMS^{TM}) and the Bjørndal criteria (score of 0–9). Parental-reported hypersensitivity was evaluated using a visual analogue scale (0–10 = no to severe pain). *Results:* Clinical variables were evaluated at baseline and three months after treatment. Thereafter, a significant decline in hypersensitivity/pain led to lower final scores in the Riva Star® group (0.40 ± 1.12, p = 0.002) than in the Duraphat® group (1.40 ± 2.20, p = 0.004). The caries arrest effect was significantly higher in the Riva Star® group (86.7%) compared to the Duraphat® group three months after treatment (13.3%, p < 0.001). In both groups, there were no statistically significant differences in the children's behavior before, during, and after treatment. *Conclusions:* Ultimately, with both fluoride therapies reducing hypersensitivity/pain significantly, treatment with 38% SDF+KI was clearly more effective in caries arrest than 5% NaF varnish after a 3-month period.

Keywords: dental caries; dentin hypersensitivity; fluoride; minimally invasive dentistry; potassium iodide; silver diamine fluoride

1. Introduction

Dentin hypersensitivity is described as short, sharp pain resulting from exposed dentin in response to external stimuli. These stimuli could be thermal, evaporative, tactile, osmotic, or chemical, and they are not attributed to any other dental disease or defect [1]. Evidence of dentin hypersensitivity (DH) prevalence in children is scarce. Reviews by Shiau [2] and Splieth and Tachou [3] reported ranges between 3 to 73% and 3 to 98%, respectively, in adults, with a higher female incidence in the former study.

Despite the limited evidence of hypersensitivity prevalence in children, this is one of the most prevalent diseases in children (early childhood caries), and it is noted to be among the common causes of hypersensitivity in pediatric dentistry [4]. Dental caries can generally be rooted to several factors, such as an imbalance in the oral microbiome and dietary habits including consumption of cariogenic food, and poor oral hygiene [5]. Early childhood caries (ECCs) is defined as the early onset of caries in young children with often rapid progression, which can eventually result in complete destruction of the primary dentition. Epidemiologically, ECCs can be defined as the presence of one or more decayed (non-cavitated or cavitated lesions), missing (due to caries), or filled surfaces in any primary tooth of a child under the age of six [6].

Although there has been a notable increase in the prevalence of ECC in industrialized countries [7], the literature concerning strategies to manage hypersensitivity in this condition is limited. Generally, dentin hypersensitivity can be treated by interrupting the neural response to pain stimuli or blocking the exposed dentinal tubules [8]. Most commonly, sodium fluoride (NaF) varnish has been traditionally used for managing hypersensitivity by occluding the causative open dentinal tubules [9]; however, this has been shown to facilitate caries arrest [10].

In 2014, silver diamine fluoride (SDF) was approved by the US Food and Drug Administration as a treatment for dentinal sensitivity [11]. It is commonly used in several countries for treating dentin hypersensitivity associated with the presence of carious lesions [12]. SDF was previously used off-label for caries arrest; however, it was recently recommended in the guidelines of the American Dental Association as a caries-arresting medicament [13].

A concern to consider regarding SDF is the black staining of the arrested carious lesions, which may result in undesirable aesthetics [14]. Despite this concern, most parents preferred this option to advanced treatment methods such as general anesthesia [15]. Applying a saturated solution of potassium iodide (KI) immediately after silver diamine fluoride application has been claimed to minimize the staining of dentin caries [16]. This is probably due to the reaction of iodide ions from the KI solution with the excess silver ions from the silver diamine fluoride solution, which forms a precipitate of silver iodide. Moreover, it was shown that dentine permeability could be reduced if potassium iodide was applied after a fluoride-containing silver diamine solution, consequently reducing dentin hypersensitivity [17]. Hamama [18] and Koizumi [19] showed positive results regarding the desensitizing and caries-arresting effect using a combined silver diamine fluoride and potassium iodide agent (38% SDF+KI; Riva Star®). However, caries arrest was reported to be poorer when potassium iodide was combined with silver diamine fluoride solution in children with caries lesions with an ICDAS score of 3 or above. On the other hand, the combination had better odds of minimizing the staining effect than solely applying silver diamine fluoride [20].

Most of the available studies refer to the prevalence, causes, and approaches used to manage dentin hypersensitivity in adults. In contrast, the literature concerning dentin hypersensitivity in children is very limited [21,22], representing a clear evidence gap concerning dentin hypersensitivity management in children, specifically that of an underlying cariological etiology. Therefore, our study aimed to evaluate the capability of 5% sodium fluoride varnish to relieve dentin hypersensitivity pain in children and to assess its impact on arresting the active carious lesions of hypersensitive primary teeth compared to treatment with 38% silver diamine fluoride and potassium iodide. The null hypothesis was that no difference would be found at three months between the two arms for the primary outcome of relieving dentin hypersensitivity pain. Moreover, as secondary outcomes, we evaluated caries arrest and compared the treating dentists' opinions on the procedures and the children's behavior in both interventions.

2. Materials and Methods

This study followed a two-arm prospective interventional design conducted in the Preventive and Pediatric Dentistry Department of Greifswald University in the period from January 2020 to March 2021. Ethics approval was granted by the Research Ethics Committee of Greifswald University on the 8th of August 2018 (No. BB 128/18; trial registration no. NCT04804423). Written informed consent was obtained from the participants' parent/legal guardian/next of kin to participate in the study to evaluate the effect of fluoride varnish and 38% SDF+KI in carious lesions.

2.1. Sample

Sample size was estimated using "G*power version 3.1" while considering the following parameters: T tests, effect size: 1, α err prob: 0.05, power (1-ß err): 0.8 and an expected mean difference of visual analog scale (VAS) values between the two comparison groups. The total sample size was found to be 28 patients. Assuming a drop-out of 10%, 30 participants were required.

2.2. Treating Dentists

Treatments were performed by six different dentists (four pediatric specialists and two post-graduate pediatric dentistry students), all of whom were briefed on the study protocol and received instructions on carrying out the interventions according to the manufacturer's guidelines.

2.3. Participant Screening, Eligibility, and Baseline Assessment

At screening, 2 calibrated dentists (kappa > 0.81) assessed, from regular clinic attendees, all eligible patients and consecutively recruited 30 healthy children who presented with active carious lesions with visible dentin (International Caries Detection and Assessment System (ICDAS) code 5) along with symptoms of hypersensitivity, and who had not used any desensitizer for at least 1 month prior to the participation date (see study diagram, Figure 1). On the other hand, children were ruled out if they presented systemic conditions requiring special dental considerations or allergies to any materials used in the study. At the tooth level, teeth that were previously restored or that clinically exhibited signs or symptoms of irreversible pulpal or periradicular pathology were excluded.

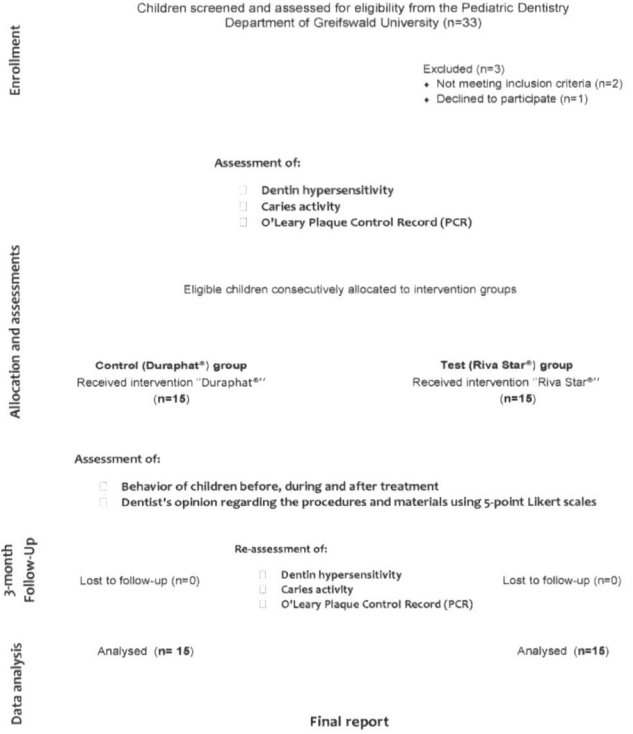

Figure 1. Study CONSORT diagram.

The eligibility examination comprised clinical assessment of active carious lesions according to ICCMS™, Bjørndal visual–tactile criteria (Table 1) [23,24], and a reported history of hypersensitivity symptoms like short-duration sharp pain in response to thermal (cold and hot drinks or food) or tactile (toothbrushing) stimuli obtained from the parent/caregiver of the child. A hypersensitivity confirmatory test using a triple-syringe air blast on the exposed surface of the carious lesion was also used to provoke a response from the patient, allocate areas with suspected dentin hypersensitivity, and eliminate possible other causes of pain [25].

Table 1. Bjørndal Criteria for Caries Activity and Severity Assessment [23].

Score	Definition
0	Sound
1	Active lesion in enamel, without cavity (bright surface with brown discoloration)
2	Active cavity in enamel (opaque enamel surface and loss of substance)
3	Active cavity in enamel (bright surface, brown discoloration, wet dentin)
4	Inactive cavity in enamel (bright surface, brown discoloration, and loss of substance)
5	Active cavity in enamel/dentin (yellow or light brown discoloration, wet dentin)
6	Inactive cavity in enamel/dentin (dark brown discoloration, hard and dry dentin)
7	Pulpal involvement or root stumps
8	Filled tooth
9	Missing tooth

The degree of pain severity was quantified via a visual analogue scale (VAS (0–10)) [26], ranging across a continuum from none (0) to a severe amount of pain (10). Moreover, assessment of the pain magnitude was verified by the accompanying parent/caregiver, mainly due to the limited communication skills due to the age of the participants, making it puzzling to quantify pain severity from the child only [27]. Following the assessment of hypersensitivity, only 1 tooth per child was included for caries activity evaluation. Following the selection of eligible teeth, a blinded second investigator (R.M.S) randomly assigned one of the eligible teeth to be included. Children's behavior before, during, and after treatment was assessed using Frankl's scale (1–4 = definitely positive to definitely negative) [28].

Consequently, eligible patients were evaluated at baseline for the following:
- Hypersensitivity pain;
- Carious lesion activity and pulp status;
- Behavior of children before, during, and after treatment;
- Dentist's opinion regarding the procedures, materials, procedure duration, and child's discomfort within the procedure in both groups using 5-point Likert scales;
- O'Leary Plaque Control Record (PCR).

2.4. Treatment Procedures and Assessment

Fluoride-desensitizing therapy was explained and discussed with the participants' parents and informed consent was obtained. Thereafter, 15 participants were consecutively allocated to receive a standard fluoride-desensitizing therapy (control arm), which included the application of 5% NaF varnish (Duraphat®, Colgate Palmolive Ltd., Guildford, UK) on the affected teeth. A second arm was set as a comparator, where an equal number of participants were consecutively enrolled under similar criteria and treated with 38% SDF+KI (Riva Star®, SDI Limited, Bayswater, Australia). Parents were always present during the treatment procedures.

The application of 5% NaF varnish followed the manufacturer's instructions: cleaned tooth/teeth, dispersion of 5–7 mm diameter drop/up to 0.25 mL of the varnish with a brush/probe/swab as aa thin layer to all affected tooth surfaces, and a recommendation not to brush the teeth or chew food for at least 1–2 h after treatment.

The silver diamine fluoride and potassium iodide agents were applied according to the manufacturer's instructions: cleaned and dried tooth/teeth, the application of a small amount of gingival barrier, when possible, and protection of the lips with petroleum jelly/cocoa without contaminating the treatment site.

In step 1, silver diamine fluoride solution (Riva Star®, SDI Limited, Bayswater, Australia) was applied using the silver brush to the treatment site, followed immediately by step 2: using the green brush provided, a generous amount of the potassium iodide solution was applied to the treatment site until the creamy white precipitate turned clear. Afterwards, all protective/isolation materials used were removed, and used brushes and capsules were discarded in accordance with local regulations.

At the 3-month recall, hypersensitivity pain (VAS), carious lesion activity (Bjørndal and ICCMS™ Criteria) and the O'Leary Plaque Control Record (PCR) were re-evaluated using the same baseline methods.

2.5. Statistical Analysis

Normality was checked for all variables using descriptive statistics, plots, and tests of normality. Means and standard deviations (SDs) were calculated for all quantitative variables, while frequencies and percentages were calculated for categorical variables. The comparison between the two study groups was performed using independent samples *t*-test for quantitative normally distributed variables (age, dt, dmft, and PCR), and Mann–Whitney U for quantitative non-normally distributed variables (mt, ft, ds, ms, fs, dmfs, percent change of PCR) and qualitative ordinal variables (lesion activity, VAS, behavior, and the dentist's opinion about the procedure). Chi-squared and Fisher exact tests were used for comparing qualitative nominal variables between the two study groups. The comparison between the baseline and follow-up was conducted using a paired *t*-test when the variable was normally distributed, and the Wilcoxon signed rank test was used when the variable was not normally distributed. The Friedman test was used to compare the children's behavior at 3 different time points (before, during, and after treatment). Binary logistic regression was performed to assess the effect of different factors on the lesion inactivity (according to Bjørndal and ICCMS™ criteria). Odds ratio (OR) and 95% confidence intervals (CIs) were calculated. Significance was inferred at $p < 0.05$. Data were analyzed using IBM SPSS statistical software for Windows (version 25).

3. Results

This prospective, comparative double-cohort study included 30 healthy children (16 males, 14 females) with a mean age of 3.67 ± 1.06, and 7.73 ± 3.16 dmft. Both cohorts consisted of 15 participants, each of which with at least one tooth with reported symptoms of dentin hypersensitivity in an active carious lesion with visible dentin (ICDAS 5) that signaled the need for a desensitizing treatment. There was no significant difference between the two cohorts regarding male/female distribution ($p = 0.57$) or dmft values ($p = 0.46$). The baseline characteristics of the participants and caries profiles are presented in Table 2.

Table 2. Sample characteristics.

		Test (Riva Star®), n = 15	Control (Duraphat®), n = 15	Total	*p*-Value
Age, mean ± SD		3.58 ± 0.95	3.76 ± 1.18	3.67 ± 1.06	0.65
Gender, n (%)	Males	9 (60%)	7 (46.7%)	16 (53.3%)	0.46
	Females	6 (40%)	8 (53.3%)	14 (46.7%)	
Caries index, tooth level, mean ± SD	dt	6.73 ± 2.43	6.87 ± 3.14	6.80 ± 2.56	0.90
	mt	0.13 ± 0.52	0.00 ± 0.00	0.07 ± 0.37	0.78
	ft	1.20 ± 1.86	0.53 ± 0.92	0.87 ± 1.48	0.54
	dmft	8.07 ± 2.79	7.40 ± 3.56	7.73 ± 3.16	0.57
Caries index, surface level, mean ± SD	ds	18.73 ± 10.48	14.40 ± 8.34	16.57 ± 9.56	0.25
	ms	0.67 ± 2.58	0.00 ± 0.00	0.33 ± 1.83	0.78
	fs	4.53 ± 7.61	1.87 ± 3.87	3.20 ± 6.09	0.57
	dmfs	23.93 ± 14.75	16.27 ± 8.96	20.10 ± 12.61	0.17

d = decay; missing; f = filled; t = teeth; SD = standard deviation.

3.1. Hypersensitivity

At baseline, the parents of two participants (13%) in the control arm (5% NaF; Duraphat®) reported severe pain (score 8, Figure 2), while moderate pain scores (4–6) dominated ($n = 5$, 33.3%, $n = 3$, 20%, and $n = 3$, 13.3%, respectively). Three months after treatment, a significant decline in pain scores ($p = 0.004$) was noticed: mostly, parents reported the absence of pain ($n = 10$, 66.7%, score 0), followed by moderate pain scores (26.6%) and mild pain (6.7%). Similarly, the assessment of pain before treatment with Riva Star® (38% SDF+KI; test arm) showed moderate pain scores on the visual analogue scale (VAS, scores 4 and 5: $n = 8$, 53.3% and $n = 7$, 46.7%, respectively). After 3 months, almost all parents reported the absence of pain in their children ($n = 13$, 86.7%, score 0; $p = 0.001$). When both interventions were compared, there was no statistically significant difference in the efficacy of both treatments in relieving hypersensitivity pain ($p = 0.31$). The assessed teeth showed vitality features and no signs or symptoms of necrosis or irreversible pulpitis.

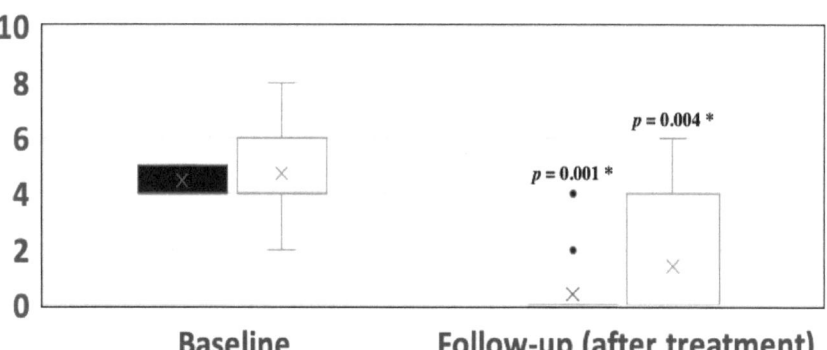

Figure 2. Pain assessment using the visual analogue scale (VAS) as reported by parents before and after treatment in the two study groups. SDF+KI: silver diamine fluoride + potassium iodide solution (Riva Star®); NaF: 5% NaF varnish (Duraphat®). * statistically significant at p-value < 0.05.

3.2. Caries Activity

At baseline, all included carious lesions in the whole sample ($n = 30$) showed visual and tactile features of caries activity during examination and were graded as ICDAS 5 and as active cavities in the enamel/dentin according to Bjørndal and ICCMS^{TM} criteria. Three months after treatment with 5% NaF varnish, caries inactivation was apparent in only two (13.3%) of the treated teeth, while the remaining teeth sustained caries activity features (12; 80%), and one tooth (6.7%) manifested pulpal involvement signs. The proportion of caries arrest in teeth treated with 5% NaF varnish to those treated with 38% SDF+KI was not statistically significant ($p = 0.10$). On the other hand, the affected teeth treated with 38% SDF+KI were re-examined using the same criteria, and 13 (86.7%) out of 15 lesions were classified as inactive cavitated lesions in the enamel/dentin. Active caries were evident in only two (13.3%) lesions at the 3-month follow-up. However, the predominance of arrested lesions over the remaining active ones was statistically significant ($p < 0.001$). Comparing both treatments, the caries arrest effect was higher in teeth treated with 38% SDF+KI ($p < 0.001$, Figure 3). No signs or symptoms of irreversible pulpal deterioration were observed.

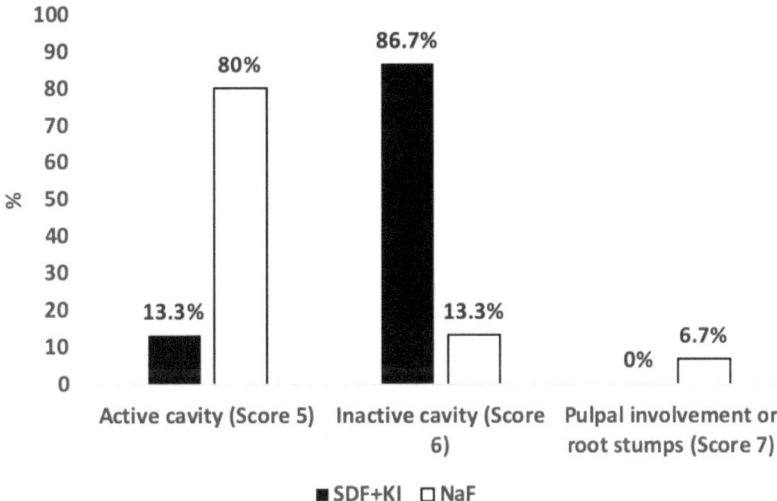

Figure 3. Activity of carious lesions according to Bjorndal criteria: post-operative assessment.

3.3. Children's Behavior

In the control arm, prior to treatment, most participants exhibited positive ($n = 6$; 40%) or definitely positive ($n = 3$; 20%) behavior during the procedure (Table 3). Immediately after treatment, negative behavior was reported in two (13%) of the participants. However, differences in behavior ratings before, during, and after treatment in this arm were not statistically significant ($p = 0.36$).

Table 3. Behavior Using the Frankl Scale Before, During, and After Treatment in the Two Study Groups.

Characteristics		Test (Riva Star®, $n = 15$)	Control (Duraphat®, $n = 15$)	Mann–Whitney p-Value
Baseline	Definitely negative	1 (6.7%)	3 (20%)	0.54
	Negative	3 (20%)	3 (20%)	
	Positive	8 (53.3%)	6 (40%)	
	Definitely positive	3 (20%)	3 (20%)	
During treatment	Definitely negative	1 (6.7%)	0 (0%)	0.29
	Negative	8 (53.3%)	5 (33.3%)	
	Positive	3 (20%)	7 (46.7%)	
	Definitely positive	3 (20%)	3 (20%)	
After treatment	Definitely negative	1 (6.7%)	0 (0%)	0.62
	Negative	4 (26.7%)	2 (13.3%)	
	Positive	6 (40%)	10 (66.7%)	
	Definitely positive	4 (26.7%)	3 (20%)	
Friedman Test p-value		0.07	0.36	

Regarding the test arm, and prior to treatment, most participants showed positive ($n = 8$; 53.3%) or definitely positive ($n = 3$; 20%) behavior. Negative behavior during treatment was noticed among eight (53.3%) children, while six (40%) children equally showed a rating of either positive or definitely positive behavior. Post-operative behavior was mainly on the positive side, with six (40%) children rated as positive and four (26.7%) as definitely positive. Only two (26.7%) participants sustained negative behavior after treatment. However, significant differences were not found between behavior ratings before, during, and after treatment in the test arm ($p = 0.07$) nor between the two study arms (Table 3).

3.4. O'Leary Plaque Control Record (PCR)

In both cohorts (Duraphat®, 44.33 ± 19.35; Riva Star®, 37.00 ± 13.07, $p = 0.23$), the mean percentages of plaque-covered surfaces were relatively high (full mouth plaque score of 20% considered as the accepted standard) before the treatment. However, there was no significant difference when plaque percentages were re-evaluated 3 months after treatment, neither in the control ($p = 0.72$) nor in the test group ($p = 0.32$). The effect of different factors on lesion inactivation was shown in the binary logistic regression model. The percent change of plaque was inversely associated with lesion inactivity (OR = 0.99; 95% CI = 0.96–1.02). Comparing inactive lesions in both groups, there was a significant difference in mean plaque percent change ($p = 0.04$); participants with inactive lesions showed almost no change in plaque percent change in the 38% SDF+KI group (0.65 ± 38.84), while there was a noticeable percent difference in the 5% NaF group (-52.08 ± 20.62).

3.5. Dentist's Opinions

Treating dentists rated the procedures as being 'very easy' or 'easy' treatments to implement (5% NaF 93.3%; 38% SDF+KI 80%). With respect to the duration of the procedures, most dentists (93.3%) considered the 5% NaF varnish application as a 'very short' or 'short' procedure to perform. On the other hand, only 66.7% of dentists classified the SDF+KI application as a 'very short' or 'short' procedure. There were no statistically significant differences between the operating dentists' opinions of both procedures undertaken ($p < 0.05$). The distribution of the data is shown in Table 4.

Table 4. Operating Dentists' Opinions about the Procedures Performed.

Questions		Test (Riva Star®) n (%)	Control (Duraphat®)	*p*-Value
Procedure Undertaken	Very Easy	4 (26.7%)	9 (60%)	0.08
	Easy	8 (53.3%)	5 (33.3%)	
	Manageable	1 (6.7%)	1 (6.7%)	
	Difficult	2 (13.3%)	0 (0%)	
	Very Difficult	0 (0%)	0 (0%)	
Materials Used in this Procedure	Very Easy to Handle	9 (60%)	11 (73.3%)	0.62
	Easy to Handle	6 (40%)	3 (20%)	
	Manageable	0 (0%)	1 (6.7%)	
	Difficult to Handle	0 (0%)	0 (0%)	
	Very Difficult to Handle	0 (0%)	0 (0%)	
Procedure Duration	Very Short/Short	10 (66.7%)	14 (93.3%)	0.17
	Time Efficient	4 (26.7%)	1 (6.7%)	
	Long	1 (6.7%)	0 (0%)	
	Very Long	0 (0%)	0 (0%)	
Child's Discomfort with the Procedure	No Apparent Discomfort	4 (26.7%)	8 (53.3%)	0.10
	Very Mild Discomfort	2 (13.3%)	2 (13.3%)	
	Mild Non-significant Discomfort	5 (33.3%)	4 (26.7%)	
	Moderate Discomfort	3 (20%)	1 (6.7%)	
	Significant Unacceptable Discomfort	1 (6.7%)	0 (0%)	

4. Discussion

This study aimed to evaluate the effect of two fluoride therapies on hypersensitive carious lesions with visible dentin (ICDAS 5) in primary teeth. For this purpose, a comparison was set between two hypersensitivity management approaches: 5% NaF (Duraphat®; control arm) and 38% SDF+KI (Riva Star®; test arm) in terms of their potential for relieving hypersensitivity and controlling the caries activity in a sample of high-caries-risk children.

The results presented in this prospective, comparative double-cohort study comprised clinical data collected at baseline and three months later. In the literature, hypersensitivity in children is barely investigated, especially when precipitated by early childhood caries (ECC). To the best of our knowledge, this is the first study to report on clinical outcomes of this kind in this age group in Europe. However, the strict listing of indications in the only registered SDF product in Europe (Riva Star®, SDI Limited, Bayswater, Australia) hindered our ability to establish a randomized clinical controlled trial. Therefore, a second arm with a matching prospective design was set to be analyzed and compared with the present study data, further allowing us to establish a study with parallel intervention and control arms and to evaluate the efficacy of the existing fluoride varnish therapy with 22,600 ppm on hypersensitive carious lesions in primary teeth [9]. In addition, to avoid selection bias, parallel recruitment of both cohorts was avoided by recruiting one full cohort first and then enrolling the second cohort. We decided by chance which cohort should be recruited first. On the other hand, treatment in the present study was performed by different qualified dentists, who were briefed and trained on the use of the product according to the manufacturer's instructions. However, only one examiner assessed the eligibility of the included subjects and evaluated the clinical outcomes at the follow-up visit. It is noteworthy to state that the evaluating examiner was calibrated on the caries classification criteria used for inclusion (ICDAS), with a substantial agreement with fellow treating dentists at a University Pediatric Dentistry department.

One of the challenges in our study was the recording and quantification of pain in children. Reliability in pre-school children's expression of pain can be problematic, since their cognitive abilities are immature with respect to accurately remembering, reporting, or quantifying pain [29,30]. With the absence of self-report, our study utilized the responses of parents/caregivers for the assessment of pain in young children. Parental perceptions have been used in oral health surveys concerning pain assessment in preschool children [31,32]. However, parental perception of pain may differ; thus, further examination was performed when severe pain or no pain was reported to avoid the misdiagnosis of irreversible pulpitis or necrosis.

Although methods such as selective electrodes or profilometers are valuable tools for quantifying surface roughness, such as in dental erosion conditions [33], and could have provided objective data on dentinal tubule blockage and reductions in hypersensitivity, our primary focus was on assessing pain perception from the patient's perspective and capturing the patient's firsthand experience of, or relief from, hypersensitivity. It is worth highlighting that these objective methods could be considered in future studies to solidify our findings.

In our study, a significant decline in hypersensitivity pain intensity was observed at the 3-month mark after the application of each fluoride therapy on the affected teeth. This downturn in pain is in agreement with findings from studies that utilized comparable pain assessment methods to the Visual Analogue Scale (VAS) to assess the effect of SDF and Duraphat® on hypersensitivity in adults [1,34]. These studies assessed the effects of fluoride therapies on a shorter-term basis. Therefore, our study's data after three months prove the sustainability of the desensitizing treatments. Another study with a comparable sample size verified the short-term effects of combining silver diamine fluoride and potassium iodide for the treatment of dentinal hypersensitivity in adults [35]. These findings could be attributed to the ability of both agents to penetrate and plug the causative open dentinal tubules. With regard to SDF, silver ions are known to leave a heavy precipitate in dentinal tubules that limits permeability [36] and calcium fluoride deposits that arise from the reaction of fluoride ions with calcium ions can also block dentinal tubules [37]. Over and above, the addition of potassium iodide over silver diamine fluoride produced a precipitate silver iodide, which has been known to contribute to the blockage of dentinal tubules [17].

The sustainability of treatment with SDF+KI can be seen as a buying-time therapy until a definitive treatment, with a lower risk than treatment under general anesthesia, can be provided. However, the long-lasting effect of SDF requires an awareness of possible factors affecting the sustainability and success of caries arrest, such as attending follow-ups for monitoring caries status and the regular removal of plaque [38].

Pertaining to caries activity, the after-effect of the application of each fluoride therapy on the affected teeth in our study cannot be overlooked. The superiority of SDF+KI over sodium fluoride varnish with regard to influencing caries arrest in primary teeth is strongly supported in the literature. Despite adopting a short-term follow-up duration, our results solidify the outcomes of similar studies in this matter [14,39,40]. Therefore, we can provide evidence of the efficiency of 38% SDF+KI over 5% fluoride varnish in a timely manner. It is our belief that the reaction precipitates of silver phosphate (Ag_3PO_4) and calcium fluoride (CaF_2) on the tooth level are responsible for enhancing caries inactivation, as the second precipitate, being responsible for the delivery of high doses of fluoride, resultantly enhances the chances of caries defeat. However, SDF mechanisms of action are diversely discussed in the literature [40–42]. Silver diamine fluoride and potassium iodide agents were used only in combination in our study. Therefore, the role of KI in caries inactivation remains unclear. In vitro studies [18,19] have shown positive results regarding the desensitizing and caries-arresting effect using combined 38% SDF+KI agents. A single study stated that SDF+KI has a higher chance of minimizing black discoloration compared with sole SDF application; however, it was also associated with a poorer carious lesions arrest rate. Yet, further clinical studies are necessary to confirm the influence of KI on caries lesions arrest [20].

On the other hand, our data revealed a potential factor impacting the probability of caries arrest following fluoride therapies. According to our analysis, the percentage change of plaque-covered surfaces is hypothesized to have an influence on the inactivation of carious lesions. However, the influence was more obvious on the inactivation of carious lesions treated with fluoride varnish than those treated with SDF+KI. Generally, disrupting the accumulation of dental plaque is known to reduce demineralizing bacterial activity and, therefore, restrain caries progression [43]. Yet, further studies with a larger sample size are necessary to affirm the influence of plaque on the inactivation of carious lesions by both fluoride therapies.

Alternately, current research has also revolved around the exploration of novel biomimetic remineralization techniques as a viable alternative to traditional fluoride-based approaches. These investigations aimed to emulate the natural mineralization process of enamel matrix and leveraging saliva-driven regeneration [44,45]. Research indicates that the use of these peptides leads to a noteworthy boost in net mineral accumulation within dental tissues [46,47]. These peptides boost mineral accumulation in dental tissues through a dual mechanism: increased mineral uptake and the prevention of mineral loss. Additionally, they stimulate the formation of new hydroxyapatite, resembling natural enamel composition [48]. However, the utilization of biomimetic nano-hydroxyapatite for enamel remineralization offers a promising alternative for preventing further demineralization at an early stage and inhibiting the onset of caries and, subsequently, hypersensitivity.

Alongside previous outcomes, our study recorded and compared the differences in children's behavior before, during, and after treatment, as well as the operators' views on the procedures in both groups.

Operators' opinions were favorable for both procedures and materials used, with no statistical significance related to any of the evaluated variables. Moreover, no significant behavioral twist was found when the children's behavior was evaluated before, during, and after treatment in both groups. Nevertheless, when dentists were specifically asked about children's discomfort with the procedures, variable discomfort rates were recorded more in SDF+KI application procedures (73.3%) than in the fluoride varnish ones (46.7%). This could be justified by the slight metallic taste and ammonia smell of the product in comparison to fluoride varnish. Overall, our operators' opinions on the acceptability of the SDF+KI application procedure agrees with a published article of dentists' opinions on the matter [49].

5. Conclusions

The analyzed data proved the efficacy of both fluoride therapies, 5% NaF varnish (Duraphat®) and SDF+KI (Riva Star®), in managing hypersensitivity in children. Moreover, our study confirmed the superior effect of combined silver diamine fluoride and potassium iodide (Riva Star®) over 5% NaF varnish (Duraphat®) in terms of arresting carious lesions with visible dentin (ICDAS 5) after three months in primary dentition. Considering the insignificant differences regarding children's behavior during fluoride application and dentists' opinions of the procedures undertaken, treatment with SDF+KI can be the favored approach to manage hypersensitivity associated with active caries lesions since it is privileged with caries-arresting potential in the short run. Obtaining parental consent for the aesthetic drawback of this treatment is essential, but it should be weighed against the alternatives, which are often restricted to more risky and invasive treatments under general anesthesia for small, uncooperative children.

Author Contributions: Conceptualization, C.H.S., R.M.S. and M.A.; investigation, M.A., M.S.M. and R.M.S.; methodology, C.H.S., R.M.S. and M.A.; project administration, M.A.; resources, R.M.S. and M.A.; supervision, R.M.S. and C.H.S.; formal analysis, R.M.S. and M.A.; writing—original draft, M.A. and R.M.S.; writing—review and editing, C.H.S., M.S.M., C.H.S., R.M.S., M.A and M.S.M. All authors have read and agreed to the published version of the manuscript.

Funding: This research received funding from the University of Greifswald and SDI Limited. The funders had no role in the study design, data collection, and analysis.

Institutional Review Board Statement: All procedures involving human participants were in accordance with the ethical standards of the institutional and/or national research committee and with the 1964 Helsinki Declaration and its later amendments or comparable ethical standards. All procedures involving human participants were in accordance with the ethical standards of the institutional and/or national research committee and with the 1964 Helsinki Declaration and its later amendments or comparable ethical standards. Approval of the local ethics committee of the medical faculty in Greifswald on the 8th of August 2018 (No. BB 128/18, trial registration no. NCT04804423).

Informed Consent Statement: Written informed consent was obtained from the participants' parent/legal guardian/next of kin to participate in the study.

Data Availability Statement: All data generated or analyzed during this study are included in this article. Further enquiries can be directed to the corresponding author.

Acknowledgments: The authors thank the patients and staff who participated in this study.

Conflicts of Interest: The authors declare that they have no conflict of interest.

References

1. Sivaramakrishnan, G.; Sridharan, K. Fluoride varnish versus glutaraldehyde for hypersensitive teeth: A randomized controlled trial, meta-analysis and trial sequential analysis. *Clin. Oral Investig.* **2019**, *23*, 209–220. [CrossRef] [PubMed]
2. Shiau, H.J. Dentin hypersensitivity. *J. Evid. Based Dent. Pract.* **2012**, *12*, 220–228. [CrossRef] [PubMed]
3. Splieth, C.H.; Tachou, A. Epidemiology of dentin hypersensitivity. *Clin. Oral Investig.* **2013**, *17* (Suppl. S1), S3–S8. [CrossRef] [PubMed]
4. Mathew, M.; Soni, A.; Khan, M.; Kauser, A.; Charan, V.S.; Akula, S. Efficacy of remineralizing agents to occlude dentinal tubules in primary teeth subjected to dentin hypersensitivity in vitro: SEM study. *J. Fam. Med. Prim. Care* **2020**, *9*, 354. [CrossRef] [PubMed]
5. Butera, A.; Maiorani, C.; Morandini, A.; Simonini, M.; Morittu, S.; Trombini, J.; Scribante, A. Evaluation of Children Caries Risk Factors: A Narrative Review of Nutritional Aspects, Oral Hygiene Habits, and Bacterial Alterations. *Children* **2022**, *9*, 262. [CrossRef]
6. Machiulskiene, V.; Campus, G.; Carvalho, J.C.; Dige, I.; Ekstrand, K.R.; Jablonski-Momeni, A.; Maltz, M.; Manton, D.J.; Martignon, S.; Martinez-Mier, E.A.; et al. Terminology of Dental Caries and Dental Caries Management: Consensus Report of a Workshop Organized by ORCA and Cariology Research Group of IADR. *Caries Res.* **2019**, *54*, 7–14. [CrossRef]
7. Çolak, H.; Dülgergil, Ç.; Dalli, M.; Hamidi, M. Early childhood caries update: A review of causes, diagnoses, and treatments. *J. Nat. Sci. Biol. Med.* **2013**, *4*, 29. [CrossRef]
8. Cummins, D. Dentin hypersensitivity: From diagnosis to a breakthrough therapy for everyday sensitivity relief. *J. Clin. Dent.* **2009**, *20*, 1–9.

9. Ritter, A.V.; Dias, W.D.L.; Miguez, P.; Caplan, D.J.; Swift, E.J. Treating cervical dentin hypersensitivity with fluoride varnish: A randomized clinical study. *J. Am. Dent. Assoc.* **2006**, *137*, 1013–1020. [CrossRef]
10. Milgrom, P.; Rothen, M.; Spadafora, A.; Skaret, E. A case report: Arresting dental caries. *J. Dent. Hyg. JDH* **2001**, *75*, 241–243.
11. FDA. Food and Drug Administration. Diammine Silver Fluoride Dental Hypersensitivity Varnish. 510(k) Premarket Notification. 2017. Available online: http://www.accessdata.fda.gov/scripts/cdrh/cfdocs/cfpmn/pmn.cfm?ID=K102973 (accessed on 20 January 2020).
12. Gao, S.S.; Amarquaye, G.; Arrow, P.; Bansal, K.; Bedi, R.; Campus, G.; Chen, K.J.; Chibinski, A.C.R.; Chinzorig, T.; Crystal, Y.O.; et al. Global Oral Health Policies and Guidelines: Using Silver Diamine Fluoride for Caries Control. *Front. Oral Health* **2021**, *2*, 685557. [CrossRef]
13. Slayton, R.L.; Urquhart, O.; Araujo, M.W.; Fontana, M.; Guzmán-Armstrong, S.; Nascimento, M.M.; Nový, B.B.; Tinanoff, N.; Weyant, R.J.; Wolff, M.S.; et al. Evidence-based clinical practice guideline on nonrestorative treatments for carious lesions: A report from the American Dental Association. *J. Am. Dent. Assoc.* **2018**, *149*, 837–849. [CrossRef]
14. Chu, C.H.; Lo, E.C.M.; Lin, H.C. Effectiveness of silver diamine fluoride and sodium fluoride varnish in arresting dentin caries in Chinese pre-school children. *J. Dent. Res.* **2002**, *81*, 767–770. [CrossRef] [PubMed]
15. Crystal, Y.O.; Janal, M.N.; Hamilton, D.S.; Niederman, R. Parental perceptions and acceptance of silver diamine fluoride staining. *J. Am. Dent. Assoc.* **2017**, *148*, 510–518.e4. [CrossRef] [PubMed]
16. Knight, G.M.; McIntyre, J.M.; Craig, G.G. Ion uptake into demineralized dentine from glass ionomer cement following pretreatment with silver fluoride and potassium iodide. *Aust. Dent. J.* **2006**, *51*, 237–241. [CrossRef] [PubMed]
17. Knight, G.M.; McIntyre, J.M.; Craig, G.G.; Mulyani Zilm, P.S.; Gully, N.J. An in vitro model to measure the effect of a silver fluoride and potassium iodide treatment on the permeability of demineralized dentine to *Streptococcus mutans*. *Aust. Dent. J.* **2005**, *50*, 242–245. [CrossRef]
18. Hamama, H.H.; Yiu, C.K.; Burrow, M.F. Effect of silver diamine fluoride and potassium iodide on residual bacteria in dentinal tubules. *Aust. Dent. J.* **2015**, *60*, 80–87. [CrossRef]
19. Koizumi, H.; Hamama, H.H.; Burrow, M.F. Effect of a silver diamine fluoride and potassium iodide-based desensitizing and cavity cleaning agent on bond strength to dentine. *Int. J. Adhes. Adhes.* **2016**, *68*, 54–61. [CrossRef]
20. Turton, B.; Horn, R.; Durward, C. Caries arrest and lesion appearance using two different silver fluoride therapies on primary teeth with and without potassium iodide: 12-month results. *Clin. Exp. Dent. Res.* **2021**, *7*, 609–619. [CrossRef]
21. de Souza-e-Silva, C.M.; Parisotto, T.M.; Steiner-Oliveira, C.; Gavião, M.B.D.; Nobre-dos-Santos, M. Oral rehabilitation of primary dentition affected by amelogenesis imperfecta: A case report. *J. Contemp. Dent. Pract.* **2010**, *11*, 71–77. [CrossRef]
22. dos Santos, M.; Brito, D.; Buzanscki, A.; Vieira, T.; Maia, L. A Minimally Invasive Approach to Manage Dental Pain in a Child with Enamel Dental Defects: 18-Month Results. *J. Bacteriol. Parasitol.* **2013**, *2*, 596. [CrossRef]
23. Bjorndal, L.; Larsen, T.; Thylstrup, A. A clinical and microbiological study of deep carious lesions during stepwise excavation using long treatment intervals. *Caries Res.* **1997**, *31*, 411–417. [CrossRef] [PubMed]
24. Pitts, N.B.; Ekstrand, K.R. International Caries Detection and Assessment System (ICDAS) and its International Caries Classification and Management System (ICCMS)—Methods for staging of the caries process and enabling dentists to manage caries. *Community Dent. Oral Epidemiol.* **2013**, *41*, e41–e52. [CrossRef] [PubMed]
25. Porto, I.C.C.M.; Andrade, A.K.M.; Montes, M.A.J.R. Diagnosis and treatment of dentinal hypersensitivity. *J. Oral Sci.* **2009**, *51*, 323–332. [CrossRef] [PubMed]
26. Gillam, D.G.; Orchardson, R. Advances in the treatment of root dentine sensitivity: Mechanisms and treatment principles. *Endod. Top.* **2006**, *13*, 13–33. [CrossRef]
27. Franck, L.S.; Greenberg, C.S.; Stevens, B. Pain assessment in infants and children. *Pediatr. Clin. N. Am.* **2000**, *47*, 487–512. [CrossRef]
28. Frankl, S.; Shiere, F.; Fogels, H. Should the parent remain with the child in the dental operatory? *J. Dent. Child.* **1962**, *29*, 150–163.
29. Versloot, J.; Craig, K.D. The communication of pain in paediatric dentistry. *Eur. Arch. Paediatr. Dent. Off. J. Eur. Acad. Paediatr. Dent.* **2009**, *10*, 61–66. [CrossRef]
30. Versloot, J.; Veerkamp, J.S.J.; Hoogstraten, J. Dental Discomfort Questionnaire: Assessment of dental discomfort and/or pain in very young children. *Community Dent. Oral Epidemiol.* **2006**, *34*, 47–52. [CrossRef]
31. Boeira, G.; Correa, M.; Peres, K.; Peres, M.; Santos, I.; Matijasevich, A.; Barros, A.; Demarco, F. Caries is the main cause for dental pain in childhood: Findings from a birth cohort. *Caries Res.* **2012**, *46*, 488–495. [CrossRef]
32. Ferreira-Júnior, O.M.; Freire, M.d.C.M.; Moreira, R.d.S.; Costa, L.R. Contextual and individual determinants of dental pain in preschool children. *Community Dent. Oral Epidemiol.* **2015**, *43*, 349–356. [CrossRef] [PubMed]
33. Paepegaey, A.-M.; Barker, M.L.; Bartlett, D.W.; Mistry, M.; West, N.X.; Hellin, N.; Brown, L.J.; Bellamy, P.G. Measuring enamel erosion: A comparative study of contact profilometry, non-contact profilometry and confocal laser scanning microscopy. *Dent. Mater.* **2013**, *29*, 1265–1272. [CrossRef] [PubMed]
34. Castillo, J.; Rivera, S.; Aparicio, T.; Lazo, R.; Aw, T.-C.; Mancl, L.; Milgrom, P. The short-term effects of diammine silver fluoride on tooth sensitivity: A randomized controlled trial. *J. Dent. Res.* **2011**, *90*, 203–208. [CrossRef] [PubMed]
35. Craig, G.G.; Knight, G.M.; McIntyre, J.M. Clinical evaluation of diamine silver fluoride/potassium iodide as a dentine desensitizing agent: A pilot study. *Aust. Dent. J.* **2012**, *57*, 308–311. [CrossRef] [PubMed]

36. Greenhill, J.D.; Pashley, D.H. The Effects of Desensitizing Agents on the Hydraulic Conductance of Human Dentin in vitro. *J. Dent. Res.* **1981**, *60*, 686–698. [CrossRef] [PubMed]
37. Thrash, W.J.; Jones, D.L.; Dodds, W.J. Effect of a fluoride solution on dentinal hypersensitivity. *Am. J. Dent.* **1992**, *5*, 299–302.
38. Sihra, R.; Schroth, R.J.; Bertone, M.; Martin, H.; Mittermuller, B.-A.; Lee, V.; Patterson, B.; Moffatt, M.E.; Klus, B.; Fontana, M.; et al. The Effectiveness of Silver Diamine Fluoride and Fluoride Varnish in Arresting Caries in Young Children and Associated Oral Health-Related Quality of Life. *J. Can. Dent. Assoc.* **2020**, *86*, 1488–2159.
39. Duangthip, D.; Chu, C.H.; Lo, E.C.M. A randomized clinical trial on arresting dentine caries in preschool children by topical fluorides—18 month results. *J. Dent.* **2016**, *44*, 57–63. [CrossRef]
40. Trieu, A.; Mohamed, A.; Lynch, E. Silver diamine fluoride versus sodium fluoride for arresting dentine caries in children: A systematic review and meta-analysis. *Sci. Rep.* **2019**, *9*, 2115. [CrossRef]
41. Mei, M.L.; Ito, L.; Cao, Y.; Li, Q.L.; Chu, C.H.; Lo, E.C.M. The inhibitory effects of silver diamine fluorides on cysteine cathepsins. *J. Dent.* **2014**, *42*, 329–335. [CrossRef]
42. Mei, M.L.; Li, Q.L.; Chu, C.H.; Yiu, C.K.Y.; Lo, E.C.M. The inhibitory effects of silver diamine fluoride at different concentrations on matrix metalloproteinases. *Dent. Mater.* **2012**, *28*, 903–908. [CrossRef] [PubMed]
43. Holmen, L.; Mejare, I.; Malmgren, B.; Thylstrup, A. The effect of regular professional plaque removal on dental caries in vivo a polarized light and scanning electron microscope study: A Polarized light and Scanning Electron Microscope Study. *Caries Res.* **1988**, *22*, 250–256. [CrossRef] [PubMed]
44. Scribante, A.; Farahani, M.R.D.; Marino, G.; Matera, C.; Baena, R.R.Y.; Lanteri, V.; Butera, A. Biomimetic Effect of Nano-Hydroxyapatite in Demineralized Enamel before Orthodontic Bonding of Brackets and Attachments: Visual, Adhesion Strength, and Hardness in In Vitro Tests. *Biomed. Res. Int.* **2020**, *2020*, 6747498. [CrossRef] [PubMed]
45. Alkilzy, M.; Qadri, G.; Splieth, C.H.; Santamaría, R.M. Biomimetic Enamel Regeneration Using Self-Assembling Peptide P(11)-4. *Biomimetics* **2023**, *8*, 290. [CrossRef]
46. Kirkham, J.; Firth, A.; Vernals, D.; Boden, N.; Robinson, C.; Shore, R.; Brookes, S.; Aggeli, A. Self-assembling peptide scaffolds promote enamel remineralization. *J. Dent. Res.* **2007**, *86*, 426–430. [CrossRef]
47. Kirkham, J.; Brookes, S.J.; Shore, R.C.; Wood, S.R.; Smith, D.; Zhang, J.; Chen, H.; Robinson, C. Physico-chemical properties of crystal surfaces in matrix–mineral interactions during mammalian biomineralisation. *Curr. Opin. Colloid. Interface Sci.* **2002**, *7*, 124–132. [CrossRef]
48. Sindhura, V.; Uloopi, K.S.; Vinay, C.; Chandrasekhar, R. Evaluation of enamel remineralizing potential of self-assembling peptide P(11)-4 on artificially induced enamel lesions in vitro. *J. Indian Soc. Pedod. Prev. Dent.* **2018**, *36*, 352–356. [CrossRef]
49. Seifo, N.; Cassie, H.; Radford, J.; Innes, N. "It's really no more difficult than putting on fluoride varnish": A qualitative exploration of dental professionals' views of silver diamine fluoride for the management of carious lesions in children. *BMC Oral Health* **2020**, *20*, 257. [CrossRef]

Disclaimer/Publisher's Note: The statements, opinions and data contained in all publications are solely those of the individual author(s) and contributor(s) and not of MDPI and/or the editor(s). MDPI and/or the editor(s) disclaim responsibility for any injury to people or property resulting from any ideas, methods, instructions or products referred to in the content.

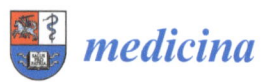

Article

Oral Health Survey in Burundi; Evaluation of the Caries Experience in Schoolchildren Using the DMFT Index

Demetrio Lamloum [1,2], Marco Dettori [2,3], Pino La Corte [4], Maria Ruth Agnoli [5], Andrea Cappai [6], Arianna Viarchi [7], Antonella Arghittu [3], Thomas Gerhard Wolf [2,8,†], Paolo Castiglia [3,†] and Guglielmo Campus [2,3,9,*,†]

1. Department of Public Health, Experimental and Forensic Medicine, University of Pavia, 27100 Pavia, Italy; demetrio.lamloum@students.unibe.ch
2. Department of Restorative, Pediatric and Preventive Dentistry, University of Bern, 3012 Bern, Switzerland; madettori@uniss.it (M.D.); thomas.wolf@unibe.ch (T.G.W.)
3. Department of Medicine, Surgery and Pharmacy, University of Sassari, 07100 Sassari, Italy; aarghittu@uniss.it (A.A.); paolo.castiglia@uniss.it (P.C.)
4. Solidarietà Medico Odontoiatrica nel Mondo (SMOM) ODV, 20143 Milan, Italy; pinolacorte@fastwebnet.it
5. Faculty of Dentistry, Universidad Alfonso X El Sabio, 28691 Madrid, Spain; magno@uax.es
6. Department of Architecture, Design and Urban Planning, University of Sassari, 07041 Alghero, Italy; a.cappai7@phd.uniss.it
7. Section of Odontostomatologic Surgery, University of Perugia, 06126 Perugia, Italy; ariannaviarchi@gmail.com
8. Department of Periodontology and Operative Dentistry, University Medical Center of the Johannes Gutenberg-University Mainz, D-55131 Mainz, Germany
9. Department of Cariology, Saveetha Dental College and Hospitals, Chennai 600077, India
* Correspondence: guglielmo.campus@unibe.ch; Tel.: +41-0316340987
† These authors share the last authorship.

Citation: Lamloum, D.; Dettori, M.; La Corte, P.; Agnoli, M.R.; Cappai, A.; Viarchi, A.; Arghittu, A.; Wolf, T.; Castiglia, P.; Campus, G. Oral Health Survey in Burundi; Evaluation of the Caries Experience in Schoolchildren Using the DMFT Index. *Medicina* **2023**, *59*, 1538. https://doi.org/10.3390/medicina59091538

Academic Editor: Gaetano Isola

Received: 20 July 2023
Revised: 3 August 2023
Accepted: 21 August 2023
Published: 25 August 2023

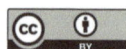

Copyright: © 2023 by the authors. Licensee MDPI, Basel, Switzerland. This article is an open access article distributed under the terms and conditions of the Creative Commons Attribution (CC BY) license (https://creativecommons.org/licenses/by/4.0/).

Abstract: *Background and objectives:* There are no data on oral health in the population of Burundi. This study aimed to describe the oral health status of schoolchildren in Burundi using the dmft/DMFT index for the first time. *Materials and methods:* The study was designed as a cross-sectional population-based epidemiological survey. The survey was designed according to the WHO methodology for oral health surveys. Oral examinations were conducted in school rooms using a dental mirror, probe, and headlight. The following characteristics of primary dentition status were recorded: decayed (d/D), missing (m/M), and filled (f/F) teeth, and the dmft/DMFT (d + m + f t/D + M + F T) index was calculated for each subject. Quantitative and qualitative variables were represented by measures of position and variability. One-way ANOVA was used to assess differences between parametric variables. Logistic regression was performed for total caries experience and gender, age groups, living area, and geographical provinces. *Results:* A total of 1902 children were examined, 1007 (52.94%) six-year-olds and 895 (47.06%) in the older group. The dmft/DMFT and subgroups were statistically significantly different in terms of age groups, living areas, and geographical regions (dmft/DMFT d-subgroup and D-subgroup $p < 0.01$), but only for DMFT for sex. The ORs estimated by logistic regression by total caries experience showed a protective effect for 12 year old subjects and those living in southern provinces, an OR of 0.52 (95%CI 0.43–0.64) and an OR of 0.26 (95%CI 0.21–0.32), respectively. *Conclusions:* Dental caries in African countries, including Burundi, remains a major problem affecting the general health and wellbeing of the population. Tackling untreated caries requires a multifaceted approach, including strengthening oral health infrastructure, promoting oral health education, providing affordable dental services, and encouraging healthier eating habits.

Keywords: caries epidemiology; children; DMFT index; Burundi

1. Introduction

In the African region, about half of the population suffers from oral diseases, most notably dental caries, periodontal disease, and tooth loss [1,2]. African countries face a disproportionate burden of tooth decay due to a number of factors, including limited access to dental care, poor oral hygiene practices, inadequate oral health education, and lack of preventive measures [3,4].

Caries prevalence has been declining in high-income countries (HICs) since the 1970s [5], but population data from many low-income countries (LICs) remain scarce. Management cost for oral diseases in LICs is skyrocketing [6]. Their impact affects quality of life, child growth, and daily activities [7,8]. The high rate of untreated caries in LICs is related to local endemic barriers, such as reduced human resources, lack of infrastructure, and poor information [9].

While numerous oral health studies have been conducted in Tanzania, Ghana, Ethiopia, Burkina Faso, and other African countries [10–14], there are limited studies on pediatric caries prevention and treatment in Burundi. The Republic of Burundi is a landlocked country in East Africa, situated in the African Great Lakes Region, to the east of the Democratic Republic of the Congo. Burundi consists of 18 regions, roughly divided into a northern hilly and mountainous part and a southern plain and with a population of 12.55 million. It has a GDP per capita of USD 221.48 [15]. According to the United Nations Development Program (UNDP), it is one of the least developed countries in the world in terms of life expectancy, literacy, and per capita income, ranking 187th out of 189th [16]. Despite the scarce economic resources and the fragmented public health system, oral health is included as a "public health problem" in the country's national agenda and the national long-term health policy (Plan National de la Santé) [17], but several constraints limit the resilience of the local health system. There is a lack of oral health promotion and primary prevention of caries in Burundi [18,19], and the economic situation poses a challenge to individuals seeking dental care. The majority of the population faces financial barriers to accessing care. The risk of catastrophic health expenditure hinders regular dental check-ups, treatment, and preventive measures [20]. Strengthening the national oral healthcare systems seems pivotal [21]. Poor dental care infrastructure, particularly in underserved areas, lack of oral health education, and insufficient numbers of dental clinics, oral health professionals, and educational interventions need to be addressed [22–26]. LICs are faced with the challenge of the increasing caries prevalence, as the upward trend is mainly due to cariogenic dietary habits, poor oral hygiene, and fragmented care services. Data are scattered, and many countries have never had an epidemiologic survey [3]. Hence, the aim of this study was to present the first survey on oral health among schoolchildren in Burundi using the dmft/DMFT index. This will allow future national integrated strategies for the provision of primary healthcare and promote cost containment in health policy planning and development.

2. Materials and Methods

2.1. Study Design and Setting

The study was conducted in Burundi (Figure 1) and was designed as a cross-sectional population-based epidemiology survey. The University of Bern (Switzerland) and the University of Sassari (Italy) collaborated in the design and implementation of the study.

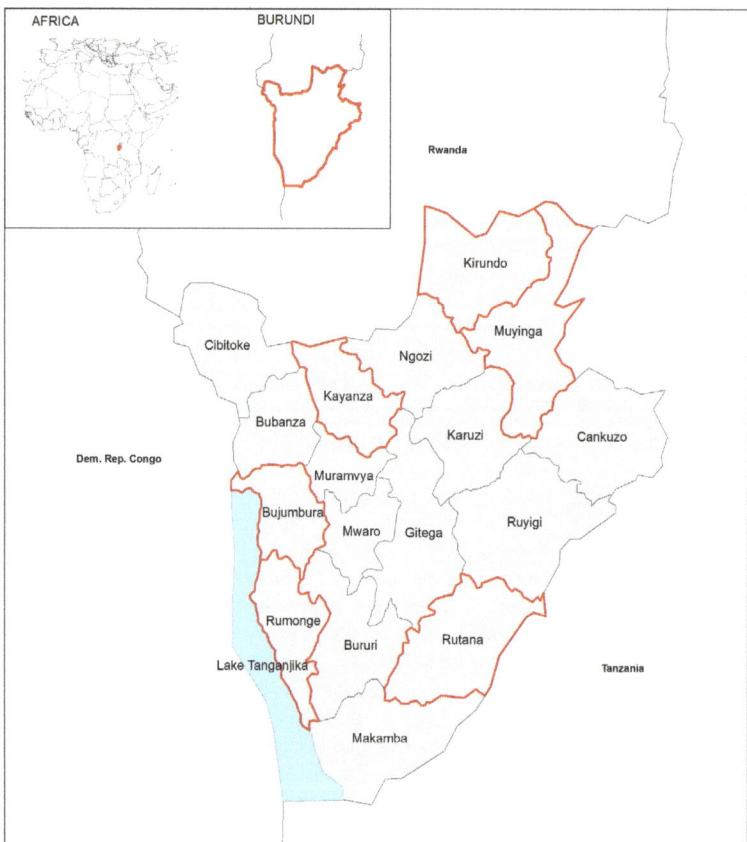

Figure 1. Geographical localization of Burundi, and areas of the study. The colored lines enclose the areas where the study took place.

2.2. Methods

Sample size was assessed using the freeware online application openepi (http://www.openepi.com version 3, (accessed on 10 July 2023)), taking into account that no data were available; therefore, an expected prevalence of 50% was considered [27,28], as the expected prevalence was within the range of 10% and 90% of the prevalence. A confidence level of 97% was used. The number returned was 471; however, as Burundi could be divided into two main areas, the sample size was doubled. This strategy resulted in a sample that was self-weighting. Each child's parents/caregivers received a leaflet explaining the aim of the study and requesting the child's participation. Only children whose parents/caregivers signed the participation form were enrolled. All the subjects belonged to two age groups: 6 and 12 years old.

The survey method was carried out after a calibration process with caries lesions detected on images and clinically by four examiners. The calibration process was carried out first on images and then on 36 subjects equally distributed between the two age groups. Intra- and inter-observer reliability was assessed using Cohen's kappa score.

The survey was designed according to the WHO methodology for oral health surveys [29]. Oral examinations were conducted in school rooms using a dental mirror, probe, and headlight. The following characteristics of the primary dentition status were recorded: decayed (d/D), missing (m/M), and filled (f/F) teeth, and the dmft/DMFT (d + m + f t/D + M + F T) index was then calculated for each subject.

2.3. Data Collection and Analysis

Data were entered into Excel (Microsoft Office, Microsoft Corporation, Redmond, WS, USA) and analyzed using STATA® 17.0 statistical software (StatCorp., Austin, TX, USA) at a statistically significant level of $p < 0.05$. Total caries experience was converted as a dichotomous variable on the basis of the dmft/DMFT index (0 = caries free; 1 = at least one tooth with a history of caries regardless of whether the active lesion tooth was extracted or filled for caries). Subjects were grouped according to whether they lived in the northern (Kayanza, Muyinga, and Kirundo) or southern (Rumonge, Rutana, and Bujumbura) regions. The living area (urban or rural) was also taken into account. Qualitative variables were described in terms of absolute and relative frequencies. Associations between categorical variables were tested using Pearson's chi-square. Quantitative variables were represented by measures of position and variability. One-way ANOVA was used to evaluate the differences between parametric variables. Multivariate analysis was performed using logistic regression for total caries experience and gender, age groups, living area, and geographical provinces. The presence of a possible effect modifier was assessed by cross-tabulation and generation of dummy variables tested by the above logistic regression analysis. The map of Burundi was retrieved from the World Atlas (https://www.worldatlas.com/maps/burundi, (accessed on 10 July 2023)) and ArcGIS software was used for geographic mapping and the shape file generation (version 10.8.2, Redlands, CA, USA).

3. Results

Intra- and inter-observer agreement, assessed using Cohen's Kappa score, was good (0.78–0.84 and 0.73–0.89 ranges for Intra- and inter-observer agreement, respectively). A total of 1902 children were examined, 1007 (52.94%) in the six-year-old group and 895 (47.06%) in the older group (Table 1).

Table 1. Demographic characteristics (sex, age groups, living area, provinces) of the enrolled sample.

	Sex		
	Males n (%)	Females n (%)	Total n (%)
6-year-olds	476 (47.27)	531 (52.73)	1007 (52.94)
12-year-olds	430 (48.04)	465 (51.96)	895 (47.06)
	Pearson $\chi^2_{(1)} = 0.11$ $p = 0.74$		
Urban	286 (46.89)	324 (53.11)	610 (32.07)
Rural	620 (47.99)	672 (52.01)	1292 (67.93)
	Pearson $\chi^2_{(1)} = 0.20$ $p = 0.65$		
Kayanza	125 (41.39)	177 (58.61)	302 (15.88)
Muyinga	247 (49.30)	254 (50.70)	501 (26.34)
Kirundo	152 (50.84)	147 (49.16)	299 (15.72)
Northern provinces	524 (47.55)	578 (52.45)	1102 (57.94)
Rumonge	149 (49.67)	151 (50.33)	300 (15.77)
Rutana	136 (45.33)	164 (54.67)	300 (15.77)
Bujumbura	97 (48.50)	103 (51.50)	200 (10.52)
Southern provinces	382 (47.75)	418 (52.25)	800 (42.06)
	Pearson $\chi^2_{(5)} = 7.70$ $p = 0.17$		

With regard to sex distribution, no statistically significant differences were observed with respect to age groups ($p = 0.74$), living area ($p = 0.65$), and regions ($p = 0.17$). Caries, dmft/DMFT, and subgroups, (Table 2, Figure 2) were statistically significantly different between age groups, living areas and geographical regions (dmft/DMFT d-subgroup and D-subgroup $p < 0.01$), but only for DMFT for sex (Figure 3).

Table 2. Caries diseases indices (dmft/DMFT) sorted by sex, age groups, living area, and provinces of the enrolled sample.

	(A) Primary Dentition					(B) Permanent Dentition		
	Males mean ± SD (range)	Females mean ± SD (range)	One-way ANOVA p-value			Males mean ± SD (range)	Females mean ± SD (range)	One-way ANOVA p-value
d	1.25 ± 2.33 (0–13)	1.33 ± 2.37 (0–16)	0.51	Sex	D	0.71 ± 1.46 (0–9)	0.89 ± 1.74 (0–12)	0.01
m	0.1 ± 0.43 (0–4)	0.09 ± 0.48 (0–6)	0.70		M	0.01 ± 0.13 (0–2)	0.01 ± 0.12 (0–2)	0.71
f	0.01 ± 0.17 (0–5)	0.00 ± 0.07 (0–2)	0.66		F	--	0.00 ± 0.03 (0–1)	--
dmft	1.35 ± 2.47 (0–13)	1.42 ± 2.50 (0–16)	0.55		DMFT	0.72 ± 1.46 (0–9)	0.90 ± 1.75 (0–12)	0.02
	6-year-olds mean ± SD (range)	12-year-olds mean ± SD (range)	One-way ANOVA p-value			6-year-olds mean ± SD (range)	12-year-olds mean ± SD (range)	One-way ANOVA p-value
d	2.28 ± 2.83 (0–16)	0.18 ± 0.67 (0–7)	<0.01	Age groups	D	0.28 ± 0.77 (0–6)	1.39 ± 2.05 (0–12)	<0.01
m	0.17 ± 0.59 (0–6)	0.01 ± 0.17 (0–3)	<0.01		M	0.01 ± 0.10 (0–2)	0.02 ± 0.15 (0–2)	0.25
f	0.01 ± 0.17 (0–5)	--	--		F	--	0.00 ± 0.03 (0–1)	--
dmft	2.45 ± 2.97 (0–16)	0.19 ± 0.70 (0–7)	<0.01		DMFT	0.29 ± 0.78 (0–6)	1.41 ± 2.06 (0–12)	<0.01
	Urban mean ± SD (range)	Rural mean ± SD (range)	One-way ANOVA p-value			Urban mean ± SD (range)	Rural mean ± SD (range)	One-way ANOVA p-value
d	1.03 ± 1.86 (0–11)	1.41 ± 2.55 (0–16)	<0.01	Living Area	D	0.35 ± 0.91 (0–7)	1.02 ± 1.82 (0–12)	<0.01
m	0.10 ± 0.42 (0–6)	0.09 ± 0.42 (0–4)	0.59		M	0.01 ± 0.09 (0–1)	0.01 ± 0.14 (0–2)	0.36
f	0.01 ± 0.22 (0–5)	--	--		F	0.00 ± 0.04 (0–1)	--	--
dmft	1.13 ± 2.02 (0–12)	1.50 ± 2.68 (0–16)	<0.01		DMFT	0.36 ± 0.92 (0–7)	1.03 ± 1.82 (0–12)	<0.01
	Northern regions mean ± SD (range)	Southern regions mean ± SD (range)	One-way ANOVA p-value			Northern regions mean ± SD (range)	Southern regions mean ± SD (range)	One-way ANOVA p-value
d	1.70 ± 2.77 (0–16)	0.73 ± 1.45 (0–10)	<0.01	Geographical regions	D	1.17 ± 1.94 (0–12)	0.30 ± 0.75 (0–6)	<0.01
m	0.10 ± 0.48 (0–6)	0.09 ± 0.42 (0–4)	0.67		M	0.00 ± 0.05 (0–1)	0.03 ± 0.19 (0–2)	<0.01
f	--	0.01 ± 0.19 (0–5)	--		F	--	0.00 ± 0.04 (0–1)	--
dmft	1.80 ± 2.89 (0–16)	0.81 ± 1.60 (0–11)	<0.01		DMFT	1.17 ± 1.94 (0–12)	0.32 ± 0.80 (0–6)	<0.01

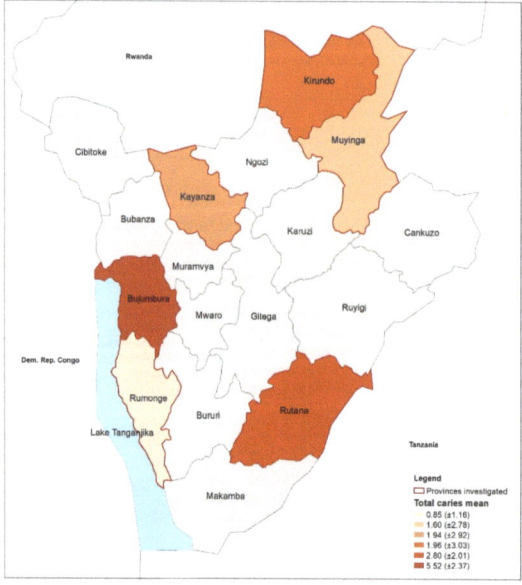

Figure 2. Total caries experience expressed as mean and standard deviation in the different areas of the study.

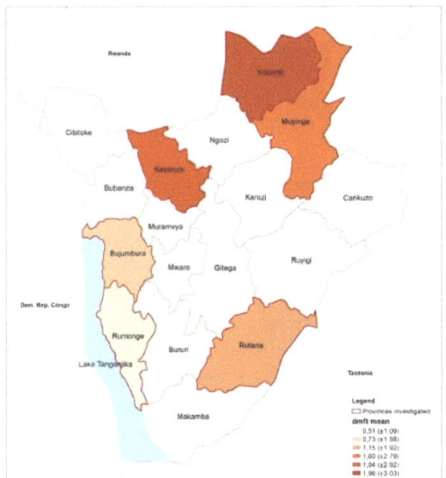
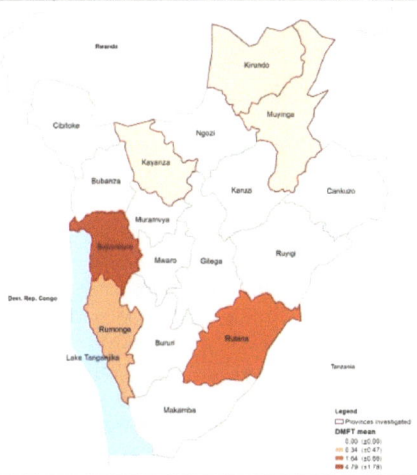

Figure 3. Caries experience in primary and permanent dentition dmft/DMFT, as the mean and standard deviation in the different areas of the study.

The difference between filled teeth (f/F) was not computed as the number of fillings was too low. The ORs estimated by logistic regression (Table 3) by total caries experience showed a protective effect for the 12 year old subjects and those living in southern provinces an OR of 0.52 (95%CI 0.43–0.64) and an OR 0.26 (95%CI 0.21–0.32), respectively.

Table 3. Logistic estimates of the model for total caries experience and gender, age groups, living area, and geographical region.

Total Caries Experience	Bivariate Analysis		Multivariate Analysis	
	OR (95% CI)	*p*-Value	OR (95% CI)	*p*-Value
Sex (*females*)	1.19 (1.00–1.42)	0.07	1.20 (1.00–1.47)	0.06
Age groups (*12-year-olds*)	0.62 (0.52–0.75)	<0.01	0.52 (0.43–0.64)	<0.01
Living area (*Rural*)	1.76 (1.45–2.14)	<0.01	1.20 (0.96–1.49)	0.104
Geographical regions (*Southern*)	0.26 (0.22–0.32)	<0.01	0.26 (0.21–0.32)	<0.01
Living area/geographical provinces (*Rural/Southern*)	0.48 (0.43–0.55)	<0.01		

The association in the logistic regression showed an effect modifier of area of residence (urban or rural) with geographical gradient. Cross-tabulation between living area and geographical area ($\chi^2 = 233.12$ $p < 0.01$) showed an inversely proportional association. A living area/geographical regions dummy variable was created, which yielded a protective OR in bivariate regression (people living in urban areas in the south had a 50% lower risk of having caries).

4. Discussion

This study provides the first data on the oral health status of schoolchildren in Burundi. A higher dmft at 6 years than DMFT at 12 years was noted. Previous studies from Ethiopia [30] and Tanzania [31] showed similar results.

The analysis showed a higher prevalence of caries in females. These data are consistent with trends in East Africa [3]. Due to premature eruption, female teeth are exposed earlier to the oral environment, bacteria, and bacterial substrates than males of the same age [32]. Dietary habits are crucial, and the exposure of females to food preparation is a direct reason, due to easier access to food and snacks outside mealtimes [32].

In the present survey, children aged 6 years were keener to develop caries in the primary dentition than in the permanent dentition at the age of 12 years. The prevalence of caries is considered age-dependent [3]. Inaccurate tooth brushing techniques are associated with a higher prevalence of caries. The highest plaque reduction was found in the 12-year-old age group and the lowest in the 6-year-olds, with no difference between the sexes [33].

Although urban populations generally report higher caries experience than their rural counterparts, a higher caries experience among children from rural areas and for the northern provinces of Kayanza, Muyinga, and Kirundo was observed. It is necessary to emphasize that the majority of the population lives in rural areas with lower per capita income. There are significant differences in the distribution of oral health services, accessibility, utilization, and outcomes between urban and rural areas in both HICs and LICs [34]. Daily consumption of processed foods and sugar is relatively higher in urban areas than in rural areas [35]. Urban populations appear to be more aware of the importance of positive dental behaviors, such as tooth cleaning and regular dental visits as oral disease prevention techniques. Rural populations also appear to be less informed about the role of fluoride in caries [36,37]. The results show that the D component is disproportionately high in all six regions. Similarly, caries management seems to be a neglected area. The F-component had a negligible contribution in our study, as almost no fillings were restored during the screening process [38–40]. Data are consistent with neighboring countries [3]. Several factors may be responsible for the high proportion of untreated caries and lack of caries treatment. The high costs associated with dental treatment and the lack of providers are important factors. Dental treatment can be costly for an average Burundian family. Implementing policies to ensure affordability and accessibility of dental services can reduce barriers to oral healthcare, as safety nets, insurance coverage, and public health initiatives are not reported [41,42].

Second, the availability and distribution of facilities and personnel represent a prerequisite for an efficient service delivery system and influence the type of services provided and the number and type of patients seen [43]. Dental shortages are often endemic on the African continent [44]. Information on the health infrastructure in Burundi is lacking, as is information on the number and location of staff. The WHO database counts 14 dentists in the country, 0.012 per 10,000 inhabitants (HICs ratio is 1:2000), according to latest data from 2018 [26]. Strengthening the dental care infrastructure through governments and international organizations will be a valid alternative impacting the caries burden, including promoting the role of mid-level providers such as dental therapists [45–48].

Parental education and income often determine access to care and preventive measures such as low-calorie, sugar-based diets, and daily use of toothpaste and toothbrushes [49]. Integrating oral health education into the national curriculum and community outreach programs can increase awareness of oral hygiene practices, the importance of regular dental check-ups, and caries prevention. Cost-effective practices at the primary care level can also have long-term results, such as sodium fluoride mouthwash for primary school children (6–12 years) and providing varnish therapy twice a year for primary school children (6–14 years).

Many African countries face several challenges in promoting healthy diets and reducing the intake of cariogenic substances [50]. In addition to poverty-related inaccessibility to healthy diets, differences in fruit and vegetable intake can be attributed to low awareness and knowledge. Although dietary intake in the Great Lakes Region is dominated by traditional local foods such as sweet potatoes, cassava, and maize, intake of so-called 'weekend foods' and Western foods (i.e., sugary drinks and snacks) is increasing rapidly [51].

At the local level, the dietary transition that has introduced soft drinks, fast foods, and Western brand names to the continent is a national phenomenon that is progressing rapidly, especially in urban areas [52]. By promoting healthy eating habits, local authorities can raise awareness of their impact on oral health and noncommunicable diseases in general, taking into account public health campaigns and regulations.

This study had some limitations. The sample of schoolchildren considered was exclusively from public schools. Public schools are publicly funded and have subsidized tuition fees, whereas private schools are privately funded and have high tuition fees. Although public schools represent the vast majority of the population, different risk factors may be associated with the more affluent individuals attending private schools. In addition, data on covariates were not collected during the screening. Information on diet, oral hygiene habits, income, and family education level is missing.

5. Conclusions

Dental caries in African countries, including Burundi, remains a major problem affecting the general health and well-being of the population. As shown by this study, untreated caries prevalence is sky-high, and caries treatments are completely absent. Providing effective measures seems a priority, and multifaceted comprehensive approaches can be a solution. By prioritizing oral health and untreated caries as part of a broader health agenda, Burundi can work toward reducing its health and social impact, particularly in more neglected areas.

Author Contributions: Conceptualization, D.L., P.L.C. and G.C.; methodology, D.L., M.D., A.A., A.C. and G.C.; validation, M.D., A.A. and G.C.; formal analysis, M.D., P.C. and G.C.; investigation, D.L., P.L.C., M.R.A., A.V. and P.L.C.; visualization, A.C.; writing—original draft preparation, D.L., M.D. and G.C.; writing—review and editing, D.L., M.D., A.A, T.G.W., P.C. and G.C.; supervision, P.C., T.G.W. and G.C. All authors have read and agreed to the published version of the manuscript.

Funding: This research received no external funding.

Institutional Review Board Statement: Consent for the study was provided by the Director General of Healthcare Supply, Modern and Traditional Medicine, Nutrition, and Registration of the Ministry of Public Health and Aids Control of the Republic of Burundi. This study did not require ethical approval.

Informed Consent Statement: Informed consent was obtained from parents/caregivers of all subjects involved in the study.

Data Availability Statement: Data are available on request.

Acknowledgments: The authors want to thank all the people in Burundi that helped to plan and run the study.

Conflicts of Interest: The authors declare no conflict of interest.

References

1. Çolak, H.; Dülgergil, Ç.T.; Dalli, M.; Hamidi, M.M. Early Childhood Caries Update: A Review of Causes, Diagnoses, and Treatments. *J. Nat. Sci. Biol. Med.* **2013**, *4*, 29–38. [CrossRef]
2. Elamin, A.; Garemo, M.; Mulder, A. Determinants of dental caries in children in the Middle East and North Africa region: A systematic review based on literature published from 2000 to 2019. *BMC Oral Health* **2021**, *21*, 237. [CrossRef]
3. Teshome, A.; Muche, A.; Girma, B. Prevalence of Dental Caries and Associated Factors in East Africa, 2000-2020: Systematic Review and Meta-Analysis. *Front. Public Health* **2021**, *9*, 645091. [CrossRef] [PubMed]
4. Lagerweij, M.D.; van Loveren, C. Declining Caries Trends: Are We Satisfied? *Curr. Oral Health Rep.* **2015**, *2*, 212–217. [CrossRef] [PubMed]
5. Bernabé, E.; Sheiham, A. Age, Period and Cohort Trends in Caries of Permanent Teeth in Four Developed Countries. *Am. J. Public Health* **2014**, *104*, e115–e121. [CrossRef] [PubMed]
6. Yee, R.; Sheiham, A. The Burden of Restorative Dental Treatment for Children in Third World Countries. *Int. Dent. J.* **2002**, *52*, 1–9. [CrossRef] [PubMed]
7. Tinanoff, N.; Kanellis, M.J.; Vargas, C.M. Current Understanding of the Epidemiology Mechanisms, and Prevention of Dental Caries in Preschool Children. *Pediatr. Dent.* **2002**, *24*, 543–551.
8. Ayele, F.A.; Taye, B.W.; Ayele, T.A.; Gelaye, K.A. Predictors of Dental Caries among Children 7–14 Years Old in Northwest Ethiopia: A Community Based Cross-Sectional Study. *BMC Oral Health* **2013**, *13*, 7. [CrossRef]
9. Petersen, P.E.; Bourgeois, D.; Ogawa, H.; Estupinan-Day, S.; Ndiaye, C. The Global Burden of Oral Diseases and Risks to Oral Health. *Bull. World Health Organ.* **2005**, *83*, 661–669.

10. Zewdu, T.; Abu, D.; Agajie, M.; Sahilu, T. Dental caries and associated factors in Ethiopia: Systematic review and meta-analysis. *Environ. Health Prev. Med.* **2021**, *26*, 21. [CrossRef]
11. Clauss, A.; Sie, A.; Zabre, P.; Schmoll, J.; Sauerborn, R.; Listl, S. Population-Based Prevalence of Oral Conditions as a Basis for Planning Community-Based Interventions: An Epidemiological Study from Rural Burkina Faso. *Front. Public Health* **2021**, *9*, 697498. [CrossRef]
12. Mbawalla, H.S.; Nyamuryekung'e, K.K.; Mtaya-Mlangwa, M.; Masalu, J.R. Dental Caries Pattern Amongst Tanzanian Children: National Oral Health Survey. *Int. Dent. J.* **2023**, *in press*. [CrossRef] [PubMed]
13. Hewlett, S.A.; Blankson, P.K.; Aheto, J.M.K.; Anto, F.; Danso-Appiah, T.; Sackeyfio, J.; Koram, K.; Amoah, A.G.B. Assessment of oral health status in a Ghanaian population: Rationale, methods, and population characteristics. *BMC Oral Health* **2022**, *22*, 67. [CrossRef] [PubMed]
14. Chikte, U.; Pontes, C.C.; Karangwa, I.; Kimmie-Dhansay, F.; Erasmus, R.; Kengne, A.P.; Matsha, T.E. Dental caries in a South African adult population: Findings from the Cape Town Vascular and Metabolic Health Study. *Int. Dent. J.* **2020**, *70*, 176–182. [CrossRef]
15. World Bank GDP per Capita (Current US$)—Burundi I Data. Available online: https://data.worldbank.org/indicator/NY.GDP.PCAP.CD?locations=BI (accessed on 6 April 2021).
16. United Nations Development Programme—UNDP Human Development Index (HDI) Ranking I Human Development Reports. Available online: http://hdr.undp.org/en/content/latest-human-development-index-ranking (accessed on 6 April 2021).
17. Burundi Ministry of Health République Du Burundi, Politique National de Santé 2016–2025. Available online: https://www.ilo.org/dyn/natlex/docs/ELECTRONIC/110854/138027/F1656560762/BDI-110854.pdf (accessed on 6 April 2021).
18. Iyer, H.S.; Chukwuma, A.; Mugunga, J.C.; Manzi, A.; Ndayizigiye, M.; Anand, S. A Comparison of Health Achievements in Rwanda and Burundi. *Health Hum. Rights* **2018**, *20*, 199–211.
19. Ahinkorah, B.O.; Seidu, A.-A.; Hagan, J.E.; Budu, E.; Mohammed, A.; Adu, C.; Ameyaw, E.K.; Adoboi, F.; Schack, T. Barriers to Healthcare Access and Healthcare Seeking for Childhood Illnesses among Childbearing Women in Burundi. *PLoS ONE* **2022**, *17*, e0274547. [CrossRef]
20. Lambert-Evans, S.; Ponsar, F.; Reid, T.; Bachy, C.; Van Herp, M.; Philips, M. Financial Access to Health Care in Karuzi, Burundi: A Household-Survey Based Performance Evaluation. *Int. J. Equity Health* **2009**, *8*, 36. [CrossRef] [PubMed]
21. Gallagher, J.E.; Mattos Savage, G.C.; Crummey, S.C.; Sabbah, W.; Varenne, B.; Makino, Y. Oral Health Workforce in Africa: A Scarce Resource. *Int. J. Environ. Res. Public Health* **2023**, *20*, 2328. [CrossRef]
22. Menegaz, A.M.; Silva, A.E.R.; Cascaes, A.M. Educational Interventions in Health Services and Oral Health: Systematic Review. *Rev. Saude Publica* **2018**, *52*, 52. [CrossRef] [PubMed]
23. Kanoute, A.; Faye, D.; Bourgeois, D. Current Status of Oral Health Research in Africa: An Overview. *Int. Dent. J.* **2020**, *62*, 301–307. [CrossRef]
24. Ramphoma, K.; Rampersad, N.; Singh, N.; Mukhari-Baloyi, N.; Naidoo, S. The Proposed Need for Integrated Maternal and Child Oral Health Policy: A Case of South Africa. *Front. Oral Health* **2022**, *3*, 1023268. [CrossRef] [PubMed]
25. Hescot, P.; China, E.; Bourgeois, D.; Maina, S.; Monteiro da Silva, O.; Luc Eiselé, J.; Simpson, C.; Horn, V. The FDI African Strategy for Oral Health: Addressing the Specific Needs of the Continent. *Int. Dent. J.* **2020**, *63*, 113–120. [CrossRef]
26. Global Health Observatory. Available online: https://www.who.int/data/gho (accessed on 12 July 2023).
27. Lwanga, S.K.; Lemeshow, S.; World Health Organization. *Sample Size Determination in Health Studies: A Practical Manual*; World Health Organization: Geneva, Switzerland, 1991.
28. Daniel, W.W.; Cross, C.L. *Biostatistics: A Foundation for Analysis in the Health Sciences*, 10th ed.; Wiley: Hoboken, NJ, USA, 2019. Available online: https://www.wiley.com/en-us/Biostatistics%3A+A+Foundation+for+Analysis+in+the+Health+Sciences%2C+10th+Edition-p-9781119625506 (accessed on 19 July 2023).
29. World Health Organization. *Oral Health Surveys: Basic Methods*, 5th ed.; WHO: Geneva, Switzerland, 2013. Available online: https://www.who.int/publications-detail-redirect/9789241548649 (accessed on 12 July 2023).
30. Teshome, A.; Yitayeh, A.; Gizachew, M. Prevalence of Dental Caries and Associated Factors Among Finote Selam Primary School Students Aged 12-20 Years, Finote Selam Town, Ethiopia. *Oral Health Dent. Manag.* **2016**, *15*, 36–41.
31. Rwakatema, D.S.; Ananduni, K.N.; Katiti, V.W.; Msuya, M.; Chugulu, J.; Kapanda, G. Oral Health in Nursing Students at Kilimanjaro Christian Medical Centre Teaching Hospital in Moshi, Tanzania. *BMC Oral Health* **2015**, *15*, 23. [CrossRef] [PubMed]
32. Ferraro, M.; Vieira, A.R. Explaining Gender Differences in Caries: A Multifactorial Approach to a Multifactorial Disease. *Int. J. Dent.* **2010**, *2010*, 649643. [CrossRef]
33. Pujar, P.; Subbareddy, V.V. Evaluation of the Tooth Brushing Skills in Children Aged 6–12 Years. *Eur. Arch. Paediatr. Dent.* **2013**, *14*, 213–219. [CrossRef]
34. Ogunbodede, E.O.; Kida, I.A.; Madjapa, H.S.; Amedari, M.; Ehizele, A.; Mutave, R.; Sodipo, B.; Temilola, S.; Okoye, L. Oral Health Inequalities between Rural and Urban Populations of the African and Middle East Region. *Adv. Dent. Res.* **2015**, *27*, 18–25. [CrossRef] [PubMed]
35. Varenne, B.; Petersen, P.E.; Ouattara, S. Oral Health Behaviour of Children and Adults in Urban and Rural Areas of Burkina Faso, Africa. *Int. Dent. J.* **2006**, *56*, 61–70. [CrossRef]
36. Kikwilu, E.N.; Frencken, J.E.; Mulder, J. Utilization of Toothpaste and Fluoride Content in Toothpaste Manufactured in Tanzania. *Acta Odontol. Scand.* **2008**, *66*, 293–299. [CrossRef]

37. Mafuvadze, B.T.; Mahachi, L.; Mafuvadze, B. Dental Caries and Oral Health Practice among 12 Year Old School Children from Low Socio-Economic Status Background in Zimbabwe. *Pan Afr. Med. J.* **2013**, *14*, 164. [CrossRef] [PubMed]
38. Simangwa, L.D.; Åstrøm, A.N.; Johansson, A.; Minja, I.K.; Johansson, A.-K. Oral Diseases and Oral Health Related Behaviors in Adolescents Living in Maasai Population Areas of Tanzania: A Cross-Sectional Study. *BMC Pediatr.* **2019**, *19*, 275. [CrossRef]
39. Fantaye, W.; Bjorvatn, K.; Bårdsen, A. The Relationship between Dental Caries and Dental Fluorosis in Areas with Moderate-High Fluoride Drinking Water in Ethiopia. *Community Dent. Oral Epidemiol.* **2004**, *32*, 337–344. [CrossRef]
40. Mwakayoka, H.; Masalu, J.R.; Namakuka Kikwilu, E. Dental Caries and Associated Factors in Children Aged 2–4 Years Old in Mbeya City, Tanzania. *J. Dent.* **2017**, *18*, 104–111.
41. Diop, M.; Kanouté, A.; Diouf, M.; Ndiaye, A.D.; Lo, C.M.M.; Faye, D.; Cissé, D. The Role of Health Insurance in the Coverage of Oral Health Care in Senegal. *J. Public Health Afr.* **2018**, *9*, 772. [CrossRef]
42. Eze, P.; Lawani, L.O.; Agu, U.J.; Acharya, Y. Catastrophic Health Expenditure in Sub-Saharan Africa: Systematic Review and Meta-Analysis. *Bull. World Health Organ.* **2022**, *100*, 337J–351J. [CrossRef]
43. Uguru, N.; Onwujekwe, O.; Ogu, U.U.; Uguru, C. Access to Oral Health Care: A Focus on Dental Caries Treatment Provision in Enugu Nigeria. *BMC Oral Health* **2020**, *20*, 145. [CrossRef] [PubMed]
44. Bhayat, A.; Chikte, U. Human Resources for Oral Health Care in South Africa: A 2018 Update. *Int. J. Environ. Res. Public Health* **2019**, *16*, 1668. [CrossRef]
45. Kaguru, G.; Ayah, R.; Mutave, R.; Mugambi, C. Integrating Oral Health into Primary Health Care: A Systematic Review of Oral Health Training in Sub-Saharan Africa. *J. Multidiscip. Healthc.* **2022**, *15*, 1361–1367. [CrossRef]
46. Friedman, J.W.; Mathu-Muju, K.R. Dental Therapists: Improving Access to Oral Health Care for Underserved Children. *Am. J. Public Health* **2014**, *104*, 1005–1009. [CrossRef]
47. Yang, Y.T.; Chen, B.; Wanchek, T. Dental Therapists: A Solution to a Shortage of Dentists in Underserved Communities? *Public Health Rep.* **2017**, *132*, 285–288. [CrossRef]
48. Edelstein, B.L. Examining Whether Dental Therapists Constitute a Disruptive Innovation in US Dentistry. *Am. J. Public Health* **2011**, *101*, 1831–1835. [CrossRef] [PubMed]
49. Schwendicke, F.; Dörfer, C.E.; Schlattmann, P.; Foster Page, L.; Thomson, W.M.; Paris, S. Socioeconomic Inequality and Caries: A Systematic Review and Meta-Analysis. *J. Dent. Res.* **2015**, *94*, 10–18. [CrossRef]
50. Abid, A.; Maatouk, F.; Berrezouga, L.; Azodo, C.; Uti, O.; El-Shamy, H.; Oginni, A. Prevalence and Severity of Oral Diseases in the Africa and Middle East Region. *Adv. Dent. Res.* **2015**, *27*, 10–17. [CrossRef] [PubMed]
51. Kiguli, J.; Alvesson, H.M.; Mayega, R.W.; Kasujja, F.X.; Muyingo, A.; Kirunda, B.; Ekirapa Kiracho, E.; Kayemba Nalwadda, C.; Naggayi, G.; Peterson, S.; et al. Dietary Patterns and Practices in Rural Eastern Uganda: Implications for Prevention and Management of Type 2 Diabetes. *Appetite* **2019**, *143*, 104409. [CrossRef]
52. Steyn, N.P.; McHiza, Z.J. Obesity and the Nutrition Transition in Sub-Saharan Africa. *Ann. N. Y. Acad. Sci.* **2014**, *1311*, 88–101. [CrossRef] [PubMed]

Disclaimer/Publisher's Note: The statements, opinions and data contained in all publications are solely those of the individual author(s) and contributor(s) and not of MDPI and/or the editor(s). MDPI and/or the editor(s) disclaim responsibility for any injury to people or property resulting from any ideas, methods, instructions or products referred to in the content.

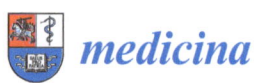 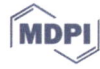

Article

Effect of Vegetable Juices on Properties of Two Resin Composites Used for Dental Caries Management

Claudia Tighiceanu [1,*,†], Elena Raluca Bulai [2,*], Oana Camelia Iatcu [2], Constantin Dulucheanu [3] and Alexandru Nemtoi [2,†]

1. Integrated Center for Research, Development and Innovation in Advanced Materials, Nanotechnologies, and Distributed Systems for Fabrication and Control, Stefan cel Mare University of Suceava, 13 University Street, 720229 Suceava, Romania
2. Faculty of Medicine and Biological Sciences, Stefan cel Mare University of Suceava, 13 University Street, 720229 Suceava, Romania
3. Faculty of Mechanical Engineering, Automotive and Robotics, Stefan cel Mare University of Suceava, 13 University Street, 720229 Suceava, Romania
* Correspondence: claudia.tighiceanu@usm.ro (C.T.); bulairaluca@usm.ro (E.R.B.)
† These authors contributed equally to this work.

Citation: Tighiceanu, C.; Bulai, E.R.; Iatcu, O.C.; Dulucheanu, C.; Nemtoi, A. Effect of Vegetable Juices on Properties of Two Resin Composites Used for Dental Caries Management. *Medicina* **2023**, *59*, 774. https://doi.org/10.3390/medicina59040774

Academic Editor: João Miguel Marques dos Santos

Received: 2 March 2023
Revised: 14 April 2023
Accepted: 14 April 2023
Published: 16 April 2023

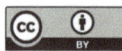

Copyright: © 2023 by the authors. Licensee MDPI, Basel, Switzerland. This article is an open access article distributed under the terms and conditions of the Creative Commons Attribution (CC BY) license (https://creativecommons.org/licenses/by/4.0/).

Abstract: *Background and Objectives*: Resin composites represent a class of materials widely used in restorative dentistry due to patient demands for better aesthetics. Colour changes in composite resins can occur due to intrinsic and extrinsic factors. Beverages, such as vegetable juices, can be some of these extrinsic factors. The purpose of this study was to investigate the colour stability and modification of microhardness of two resin composites before and after immersion in different vegetable juices. *Materials and Methods*: The colour of two resin composite materials (Gradia Direct Anterior-shade A2 and Valux Plus—shade A2) was measured before and after immersion in four different solutions: distilled water (as control), beetroot, carrot, and tomato juice. Colour values (L *, a *, b *) were measured over a white background with a colorimeter, using the CIE L *a *b * system. Colour change values were calculated after 1, 3, 5, and 7 days of immersion. Microhardness measurements were taken before and after seven days immersion in test media. Repeated measures analysis of variance (ANOVA) and independent *t*-tests were applied for statistical analysis. *Results:* All vegetable juices produced statistically different discolouration after immersion for 7 days ($p < 0.05$). Tomato juice produced the most discolouration for the Gradia Direct specimens, whereas beetroot juice and carrot juice produced the most discolouration for the Valux Plus specimens. Microhardness of the materials immersed for 7 days in vegetable juices was reduced compared to the ones immersed in distilled water. *Conclusions:* Vegetable juices, immersion time, and dental resin composites are significant factors that may affect colour stability and microhardness of composite resins.

Keywords: resin composites; colour change; vegetable juices; caries management; microhardness

1. Introduction

Dental restorative materials are used to replace a decayed portion of tooth structure due to dental cavities, dental traumas, or tooth wear, and UV light is commonly used by dentists to cure fillings [1]. Among these materials, the use of composite resins has increased recently due to increasing demands for aesthetic restorations. Besides the aesthetic appearance, physical and mechanical properties of these materials are also of great importance. Any aesthetic restorative material must simulate tooth surface texture and its natural colour and also maintain these characteristics for long periods of time. However, discolouration of dental materials remains a major problem for their long-term use [2–7].

Discolouration of restorations can be caused by two factors: extrinsic and intrinsic. Intrinsic staining is permanent and can be related to the matrix, type, and amount of filler; photoinitiator system; and polymerization degree (conversion rate) of the composite resins.

Extrinsic factors include surface stains, accumulation of plaque, superficial degradation, or a slight penetration of staining agents in the superficial layers of dental materials which can lead to alterations of surface or subsurface colour. Moreover, externally induced discolouration can be associated with surface integrity and surface roughness, which is related to the finishing and polishing technique [4–10].

Dental materials are inevitably exposed to food and drinks which may cause a colour change and may affect the aesthetic and physical properties. The degree of discolouration is affected by oral hygiene, smoking, and eating–drinking habits. Previous studies on colour stability and surface properties of composites have shown that different beverages, such as coffee, tea, red wine, juices, and carbonated drinks, may affect not only the aesthetic but also the physical properties of composite resins, thereby undermining the quality of the restoration. The effect of beverages on the properties of composite resins may also be directly related to the amount and frequency of their intake [4,8,9,11–16]. Several studies suggest that nanohybrid composites do not exhibit superior stain resistance compared to microhybrid composites when immersed in different beverages. Therefore, the chosen materials for this study were a microhybrid and a hybrid composite [15–17]. Consumption of 100% fruit juice beverages is an easy way to increase the nutrients in the diets of adults and children. Besides fruit juices, vegetable juices are also commonly consumed. Juices (even vegetable juices) contain naturally occurring acids that can lead to tooth decay, dental erosion, or colour changes. Among vegetable juices, beetroot, carrot, and tomato juices were selected as they are frequently introduced into adults' and children's diets; are known to be high in antioxidants, easily accessible, and affordable; and have a strong potential to stain tooth restorative materials [18].

The aim of this study was to evaluate the effects of immersion in different vegetable juices (beetroot, carrot, and tomato juices) on the colour and microhardness of two resin-based composite materials. The null hypotheses tested were: (i) vegetable juices have no effect on the colour stability of the resin composites chosen for the study at different times, and (ii) there are no differences in microhardness between resin composites immersed in vegetable juices for 7 days and the ones immersed in distilled water.

2. Materials and Methods

2.1. Materials and Sample Preparation

Two resin composite materials were used in this study: micro-filled hybrid resin composite Gradia Direct Anterior, shade A2 (GC Corporation, Tokyo, Japan, Lot number 2102191) and hybrid resin composite Valux Plus, shade A2 (3M ESPE, USA, Lot number NE88327). The light source used to light cure the specimens was Dental Curing Light (Curing Pen, Eighteeth, Changzhou Sifary Medical Technology Co., Ltd., Changzhou, China). The storage environments were commercially available 100% vegetable juices (beetroot juice, carrot juice, and tomato juice) (Josef Polz, Garching, Germany), and distilled water was used as the control.

A total of 72 samples (36 samples for each material), 14 ± 0.1 mm diameter and 1.5 ± 0.1 mm thick, were prepared using a circular mould held between two glass slides. A 2 kg weight was placed on top for 1 min to facilitate uniformity of the sample. Samples were cured for 20 s on each side (40 s in total) with a light-curing device set at 1500 mW/cm^2 at a 2 mm distance. After polymerization, the samples were removed from the mould and polished on one side using KENDA C.G.I., Polishers for Composites, Compomers, and Glass-Ionomers Polishers, Coarse. The final thickness of the polished specimens was 1.4 ± 0.1 mm, which was verified by a micrometre (Mitutoyo, Kawasaki, Japan).

After preparation, all samples were stored in distilled water at 37 °C for 24 h, for water absorption and completion of the polymerisation process, in proximity to oral conditions, using a Forced-Air Drying Oven (BOV V136F, Biobase, Jinan, China). Specimens of each type of composite were then randomly divided into 4 subgroups (n = 9) [9]: group 1 to be immersed in distilled water (which acted as a control group), group 2 to be immersed in beetroot juice, group 3 to be immersed in carrot juice, and group 4 to be immersed in tomato juice, for a total period of seven days at 37 °C. Baseline measurements were made following 24 h immersion in distilled water.

The pH of each beverage was measured before immersion with a pH meter (SevenCompact S210, Mettler–Toledo GmbH, Greifensee, Switzerland) (pH distilled water 6.58 ± 0.1, beetroot juice 4.34 ± 0.06, carrot juice 4.42 ± 0.02, tomato juice 4.26 ± 0.04). Beverages were used at a temperature of about 4 °C, and they were replaced daily to prevent possible interactions/bacterial adhesion.

2.2. Colour Stability Testing

The colour was evaluated on the polished side of the specimens using a colorimeter (Chroma Meter CR400, Konica Minolta, Tokyo, Japan) against a white background using the Commission International de I'Eclairage CIE (L *a *b *) colour system [5,8]. The colour was measured before being immersed in beverages as a baseline and also after immersion for 1, 3, 5, and 7 days, respectively. At each time point, specimens were rinsed with distilled water for 20 s after being removed from the solution and blotted dry with absorbent paper. The overall colour change ΔE^* was calculated from the single colour values L^*, a^*, and b^*, according to Equation (1) [4,9,12]:

$$\Delta E^* = [(\Delta L^*)^2 + (\Delta a^*)^2 + (\Delta b^*)^2]^{1/2} \tag{1}$$

ΔL^* describes the differences in brightness, Δa^* stands for the changes on the red–green axis, and Δb^* depicts the shifting on the yellow–blue axis.

As previously described in the literature, the following scale was used to classify the resulting colour difference values (ΔE): a difference below 2.0 units in the CIE colour space was classified as unnoticeable, between 2.1 and 3.5 units as slightly perceptible, between 3.6 and 5.0 units as clearly perceptible, and 5.1 units or above as pronounced [11].

2.3. Microhardness Measurement

Vickers microhardness values were measured by testing four samples from each group [19] before and after 7 days of immersion in the solutions, using a MicroHardness Tester (DuraScan 70, Emco Prüfmaschinen-Test GmbH, Kuchl, Austria). For every sample, three indentations were made, each being no closer than 0.5 mm to the adjacent indentation (EN ISO 6507-1:2018), and the test load of the Vickers indenter was 4.9 N (0.5 kgf). The two diagonal lengths of each indentation were measured by a 40× magnification built-in scale microscope and were converted into a microhardness value (HV) using the following equation: $HV = 1.854 \, P/d^2$, where HV is microhardness in kgf/mm^2, P is the load in kgf, and d is the average length of the diagonals in mm.

2.4. Statistical Analysis

Data were analysed using SPSS software version 20. Descriptive statistics, including mean, standard deviation of mean, and minimum and maximum values, were calculated for each group. An independent t-test was used to compare the data after immersion in vegetable juices and water. To evaluate the differences between the discolouration observed at different immersion time points, repeated measures ANOVA was used. In the present study, $p \leq 0.05$ was considered as the level of significance. An independent t-test was used to compare the data on microhardness of the composite materials following 7 days immersion in vegetable juices and water.

3. Results

3.1. Effect of Vegetable Juices on Colour Stability of Resin Composites

The results for the colour measurements of the tested samples at different time points of immersion and in the different vegetable juices are shown in Tables S1 and S2, which can be found in the Supplementary Material, in Table 1, and in Figures 1 and 2.

Table 1. *p*-values for independent *t*-test (for comparison of ΔE * for both materials at different time points).

	Day 1	Day 3	Day 5	Day 7
Beetroot juice	0.037 *	<0.001 *	0.011 *	0.004 *
Carrot juice	0.113	0.010 *	0.004 *	0.031 *
Tomato juice	0.540	0.235	0.536	0.260

* Indicates significant difference.

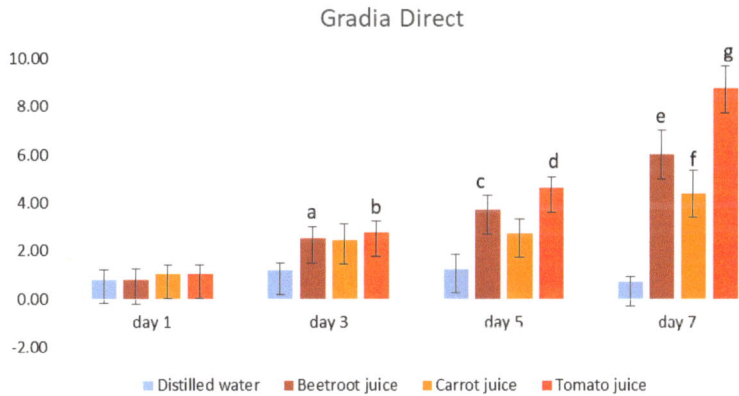

Figure 1. Colour change (mean values ± standard error of mean) for Gradia Direct samples. A lowercase letter indicates a statistical difference between the mean discolouration of samples immersed in distilled water and that of samples immersed in vegetable juice at each time point (e.g., "a" indicates a statistical difference between the mean discolouration of samples immersed in distilled water and that of samples immersed in beetroot juice for 3 days).

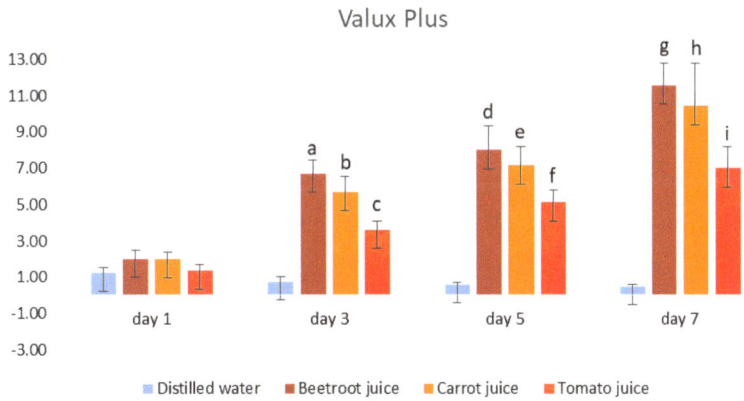

Figure 2. Colour change (mean values ± standard error of mean) for Valux Plus samples. A lowercase letter indicates a statistical difference between the mean discolouration of samples immersed in distilled water and that of samples immersed in vegetable juice at each time point (e.g., "b" indicates a statistical difference between the mean discolouration of samples immersed in distilled water and that of samples immersed in carrot juice for 3 days).

For Gradia Direct samples, imperceptible differences with ΔE < 2.0 were noted after immersion in water at all time points and after immersion in all vegetable juices for 1 day. Slightly perceptible differences with ΔE between 2.1 and 3.5 were recorded for samples immersed in all vegetable juices for 3 days and also for samples immersed in carrot juice for 5 days. Clearly perceptible differences with ΔE between 3.6 and 5.0 were observed for beetroot and tomato juices at day 5. A pronounced colour difference was noted only at day 7 for samples immersed in beetroot juice and tomato juice. The highest value of ΔE was recorded from tomato juice as the staining liquid after 7 days of immersion (ΔE = 8.74 ± 0.92).

The statistical analysis of mean colour change ΔE of Gradia Direct samples immersed in vegetable juices versus control (samples immersed in distilled water) for each time point is presented in Table S1. The results showed a statistical difference between the mean discolouration of samples immersed in distilled water and samples immersed in beetroot and tomato juices for 3 days and 5 days, respectively, and also samples immersed in all vegetable juices for 7 days ($p < 0.05$).

A statistical analysis of mean discolouration of Gradia Direct samples immersed in vegetable juices at consecutive time points of immersion was also conducted using repeated measures ANOVA. In beetroot juice, statistically significant differences were observed between day 3 and day 5 ($p = 0.012$) and between day 5 and day 7 ($p = 0.037$). In carrot juice, statistically significant differences were observed between day 3 and day 5 ($p = 0.013$) and between day 5 and day 7 ($p = 0.002$). In tomato juice, statistically significant differences were observed between day 3 and day 5 ($p = 0.001$) and between day 5 and day 7 ($p < 0.001$).

For the Valux Plus samples, similar to Gradia Direct, imperceptible differences with ΔE < 2.0 were noted after immersion in water at all time points and after immersion in all vegetable juices for 1 day. For samples immersed in beetroot juice for 1 day, the average ΔE was 2.01, a value close to the threshold and therefore considered an imperceptible difference. Starting day 3, the effect of vegetable juice on the colour of the samples was more pronounced for the Valux Plus than for Gradia Direct ones. For the samples immersed in beetroot and carrot juices, ΔE was higher than 5.0, and the samples immersed in tomato juice for 3 days showed a clearly perceptible difference with ΔE = 3.60. A pronounced colour difference was noted after 5 days of immersion and also after 7 days for all Valux Plus samples immersed in vegetable juices, with the highest value of ΔE being recorded from beetroot juice as the staining liquid after 7 days of immersion (ΔE = 11.53 ± 1.27).

The results of the independent t-test showed a statistical difference between the mean discolouration of samples immersed in distilled water and samples immersed in all vegetable juices for 3, 5, and 7 days, respectively ($p < 0.05$).

The mean discolouration of Valux Plus samples immersed in vegetable juices was statistically analysed over the 7 days by repeated measures ANOVA, between consecutive time points. In beetroot juice, statistically significant differences were observed between day 1 and day 3 ($p < 0.001$) and between day 5 and day 7 ($p = 0.031$). In carrot juice, statistically significant differences were observed between day 1 and day 3 ($p < 0.001$). In tomato juice, differences in the colour of the material were observed between day 1 and day 3 ($p < 0.001$) and between day 3 and day 5 ($p = 0.007$).

An independent t-test was used to compare the mean discolouration of Gradia Direct and Valux Plus samples exposed to the same vegetable juice at each time point to see if these materials were affected differently by the test media (Table 1). As shown in Table 1, no significant difference was found between the mean discolouration of Gradia Direct and Valux Plus samples immersed in tomato juice at any time point and for those immersed in carrot juice for 1 day ($p > 0.05$). At 3-, 5-, and 7-days immersion time in carrot juice, results showed a significant difference between the materials ($p < 0.05$). Beetroot juice appeared to be the only vegetable juice tested that affected the two materials differently, with a significant difference being observed at all time points ($p < 0.05$).

3.2. Effect of Vegetable Juices on Microhardness of Resin Composites

Microhardness measurements were taken before and after seven days of immersion in test media and reported as mean ± standard error of mean. Microhardness measurements taken before immersion in vegetable juices were 40 ± 0.16 for Gradia Direct and 129 ± 0.55 for Valux Plus samples. Microhardness results for Gradia Direct and Valux Plus samples after seven days of immersion in vegetable juices are reported in Table 2. Results showed that the microhardness of Valux Plus samples was greater than that of Gradia Direct samples. For both materials, microhardness values reduced slightly in all the groups following exposure to vegetable juices compared to those immersed in water. An independent t-test was used to evaluate the effect of beverages on microhardness. For both materials, statistically significant differences in microhardness were observed after seven days of immersion in all three types of vegetable juice when compared to those immersed in water (Table 2).

Table 2. HV microhardness (Mean ± Standard Error of Mean) of Gradia Direct and Valux Plus samples after seven days of immersion in test media.

	Gradia Direct		Valux Plus	
	Mean ± SEM	p Value	Mean ± SEM	p Value
Water	39.76 ± 1.20	-	121.33 ± 2.39	-
Beetroot juice	38.57 ± 0.97	0.014 *	119.17 ± 1.27	0.013 *
Carrot juice	37.96 ± 1.44	0.003 *	119.00 ± 1.21	0.008 *
Tomato juice	37.60 ± 0.61	<0.001 *	118.75 ± 1.22	0.004 *

* Indicates significant difference.

The percentage variation in microhardness of samples immersed for seven days in vegetable juice compared with those immersed in water was evaluated by Equation (2).

$$\text{Percentage variation in microhardness} = (\text{Microhardness in water} - \text{Microhardness in juice})/\text{Microhardness in water} \times 100 \quad (2)$$

The results obtained are presented in Figure 3. The standard fraction change in microhardness for both materials followed the same pattern, increasing from beetroot juice to carrot juice and tomato juice. Percentage variation in microhardness appeared to be more pronounced for Gradia Direct samples compared with Valux Plus samples, and tomato juice seemed to have a greater effect compared to the other two vegetable juices.

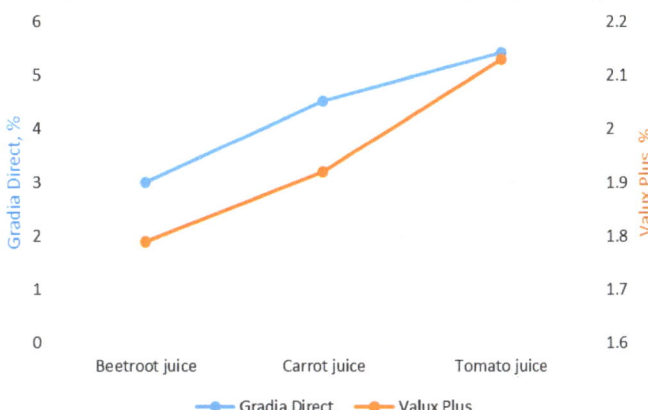

Figure 3. Percentage variation in microhardness for Gradia Direct and Valux Plus samples.

4. Discussion

Discolouration of dental restorative materials constitutes a continuous challenge in dentistry and can be a reason for the replacement of dental restorations, especially in aesthetic areas. This process concerns both patients and dentists and is time- and money-consuming.

Colour changes can be evaluated using a visual method, which is subjective and thus of low reproducibility, or by instrumental techniques, which give objective and statistically utilizable results. In dentistry, colour measurement devices are generally utilised, and the Commission International de I'Eclairage CIE (L *a *b *) colour system is used to determine the colour differences or changes.

The results of this study indicated that colour changes varied based on the type of resin composite, time of immersion, and staining liquid. After immersion in vegetable juices, it was observed that the colour differences (ΔE) increased for both resin composites over the experimental period, regardless of staining solution; the most intense colour change occurred after seven days.

Among all the vegetable juices tested, the largest colour change for Gradia Direct samples was observed in tomato juice, followed by beetroot and carrot juices. The largest colour change for Valux Plus samples was seen in beetroot juice, followed by carrot juice and tomato juice. When comparing the two materials, microhybrid Gradia Direct samples generally exhibited the least colour changes, except for samples immersed in tomato juice for seven days where a ΔE value of 8.74 ± 0.92 was recorded compared with $\Delta E = 6.95 \pm 1.22$ for Valux Plus. In this study, pH measurements showed similar values for all vegetable juices, and they were in the acidic region.

The colour changes in resin composites after immersion in various liquid beverages has been a subject of great interest in many studies. Factors that influence colour changes can be attributed both to beverages (colourants, pH) and dental materials (composition, properties). Acidic foods and beverages may induce discolouration by affecting surface integrity. The staining susceptibility of resin composites might be related to their degree of water sorption and the hydrophilicity of the matrix resin. The absorption and adsorption of colourants with different polarities, found in different beverages, on the surface of resin composites have also been proposed as potential factors. Additionally, it has been suggested that silanisation of filler particles plays an important role in discolouration due to the fact that silane has high water absorption levels [4,8,9,11,13].

Our findings showed that Valux Plus had generally lower colour stability compared to Gradia Direct. Differences in resin matrix and filler compositions could be factors that determined different discolourations of the two composites. The resin matrix of the Valux Plus product contains Bisphenol A Diglycidyl Ether Dimethacrylate (BISGMA), Triethylene Glycol Dimethacrylate (TEGDMA) and silane treated ceramic, which are considered vulnerable to staining due to their increased hydrophilicity [20,21]. These composites have zirconia/silica fillers [22,23], which may have a porosity that facilitates colourant penetration. These results are in agreement with previous studies that have reported that products that contain similar components in the matrix and fillers, as in Valux Plus, were prone to staining and discolouration [8].

Immersion in different test media can result in the degradation of the matrix and fillers of resin composites, to some extent. Surface hardness can be used as a predictor of the wear resistance of a material [24]. The wear behaviour of the composite resins can be affected not only by the type, size, and distribution of the filler, but also by the matrix and the bonding strength between the matrix and filler. In addition, by increasing the volume fraction of the filler, the wear loss decreases [25,26]. Pre-polymerized fillers have a lower hardness than silica and zirconia mineral fillers [27].

Previous studies have reported that the filler fraction for Gradia Direct is 73% by weight (64% by volume), containing silica and pre-polymerized fillers (average particle size 0.85 μm), and for Valux–Plus, it is 85% by weight (66% by volume), containing zirconia–silica fillers (particle size 0.6–1 μm) [22,23]. In this study, microhardness values for Gradia Direct samples were found to be significantly lower than for Valux Plus samples. This

3.2. Effect of Vegetable Juices on Microhardness of Resin Composites

Microhardness measurements were taken before and after seven days of immersion in test media and reported as mean ± standard error of mean. Microhardness measurements taken before immersion in vegetable juices were 40 ± 0.16 for Gradia Direct and 129 ± 0.55 for Valux Plus samples. Microhardness results for Gradia Direct and Valux Plus samples after seven days of immersion in vegetable juices are reported in Table 2. Results showed that the microhardness of Valux Plus samples was greater than that of Gradia Direct samples. For both materials, microhardness values reduced slightly in all the groups following exposure to vegetable juices compared to those immersed in water. An independent t-test was used to evaluate the effect of beverages on microhardness. For both materials, statistically significant differences in microhardness were observed after seven days of immersion in all three types of vegetable juice when compared to those immersed in water (Table 2).

Table 2. HV microhardness (Mean ± Standard Error of Mean) of Gradia Direct and Valux Plus samples after seven days of immersion in test media.

	Gradia Direct		Valux Plus	
	Mean ± SEM	p Value	Mean ± SEM	p Value
Water	39.76 ± 1.20	-	121.33 ± 2.39	-
Beetroot juice	38.57 ± 0.97	0.014 *	119.17 ± 1.27	0.013 *
Carrot juice	37.96 ± 1.44	0.003 *	119.00 ± 1.21	0.008 *
Tomato juice	37.60 ± 0.61	<0.001 *	118.75 ± 1.22	0.004 *

* Indicates significant difference.

The percentage variation in microhardness of samples immersed for seven days in vegetable juice compared with those immersed in water was evaluated by Equation (2).

$$\text{Percentage variation in microhardness} = (\text{Microhardness in water} - \text{Microhardness in juice})/\text{Microhardness in water} \times 100 \quad (2)$$

The results obtained are presented in Figure 3. The standard fraction change in microhardness for both materials followed the same pattern, increasing from beetroot juice to carrot juice and tomato juice. Percentage variation in microhardness appeared to be more pronounced for Gradia Direct samples compared with Valux Plus samples, and tomato juice seemed to have a greater effect compared to the other two vegetable juices.

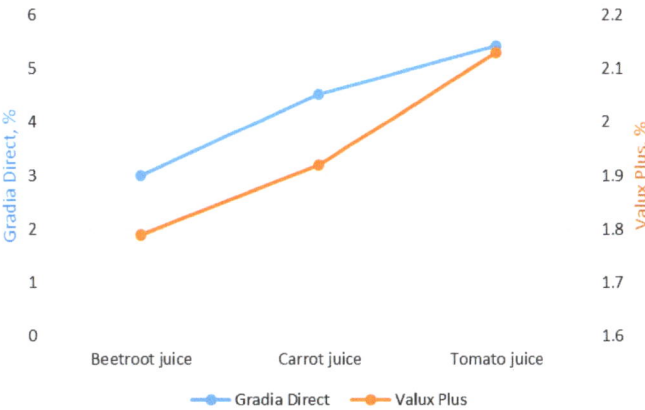

Figure 3. Percentage variation in microhardness for Gradia Direct and Valux Plus samples.

4. Discussion

Discolouration of dental restorative materials constitutes a continuous challenge in dentistry and can be a reason for the replacement of dental restorations, especially in aesthetic areas. This process concerns both patients and dentists and is time- and money-consuming.

Colour changes can be evaluated using a visual method, which is subjective and thus of low reproducibility, or by instrumental techniques, which give objective and statistically utilizable results. In dentistry, colour measurement devices are generally utilised, and the Commission International de I'Eclairage CIE (L *a *b *) colour system is used to determine the colour differences or changes.

The results of this study indicated that colour changes varied based on the type of resin composite, time of immersion, and staining liquid. After immersion in vegetable juices, it was observed that the colour differences (ΔE) increased for both resin composites over the experimental period, regardless of staining solution; the most intense colour change occurred after seven days.

Among all the vegetable juices tested, the largest colour change for Gradia Direct samples was observed in tomato juice, followed by beetroot and carrot juices. The largest colour change for Valux Plus samples was seen in beetroot juice, followed by carrot juice and tomato juice. When comparing the two materials, microhybrid Gradia Direct samples generally exhibited the least colour changes, except for samples immersed in tomato juice for seven days where a ΔE value of 8.74 ± 0.92 was recorded compared with $\Delta E = 6.95 \pm 1.22$ for Valux Plus. In this study, pH measurements showed similar values for all vegetable juices, and they were in the acidic region.

The colour changes in resin composites after immersion in various liquid beverages has been a subject of great interest in many studies. Factors that influence colour changes can be attributed both to beverages (colourants, pH) and dental materials (composition, properties). Acidic foods and beverages may induce discolouration by affecting surface integrity. The staining susceptibility of resin composites might be related to their degree of water sorption and the hydrophilicity of the matrix resin. The absorption and adsorption of colourants with different polarities, found in different beverages, on the surface of resin composites have also been proposed as potential factors. Additionally, it has been suggested that silanisation of filler particles plays an important role in discolouration due to the fact that silane has high water absorption levels [4,8,9,11,13].

Our findings showed that Valux Plus had generally lower colour stability compared to Gradia Direct. Differences in resin matrix and filler compositions could be factors that determined different discolourations of the two composites. The resin matrix of the Valux Plus product contains Bisphenol A Diglycidyl Ether Dimethacrylate (BISGMA), Triethylene Glycol Dimethacrylate (TEGDMA) and silane treated ceramic, which are considered vulnerable to staining due to their increased hydrophilicity [20,21]. These composites have zirconia/silica fillers [22,23], which may have a porosity that facilitates colourant penetration. These results are in agreement with previous studies that have reported that products that contain similar components in the matrix and fillers, as in Valux Plus, were prone to staining and discolouration [8].

Immersion in different test media can result in the degradation of the matrix and fillers of resin composites, to some extent. Surface hardness can be used as a predictor of the wear resistance of a material [24]. The wear behaviour of the composite resins can be affected not only by the type, size, and distribution of the filler, but also by the matrix and the bonding strength between the matrix and filler. In addition, by increasing the volume fraction of the filler, the wear loss decreases [25,26]. Pre-polymerized fillers have a lower hardness than silica and zirconia mineral fillers [27].

Previous studies have reported that the filler fraction for Gradia Direct is 73% by weight (64% by volume), containing silica and pre-polymerized fillers (average particle size 0.85 μm), and for Valux–Plus, it is 85% by weight (66% by volume), containing zirconia–silica fillers (particle size 0.6–1 μm) [22,23]. In this study, microhardness values for Gradia Direct samples were found to be significantly lower than for Valux Plus samples. This could be associated with the lower amount of filling in Gradia Direct compared with Valux Plus samples, and also with the type of filling, which would be in agreement with previous studies where composites with the highest filler by volume exhibited the highest hardness.

The pH is a very valuable indicator of the body's health, starting from the oral cavity. Good oral health involves maintaining an environment of the mouth near a neutral pH. An acidic pH in the oral cavity contributes to dental erosion. Previous studies have shown that some acidic foods and beverages can cause surface degradation and reduce surface hardness of restorative dental materials [19,28–31]. In this study, both tested resin composites registered a slight decrease in microhardness after one week immersion in juices, compared with samples immersed in distilled water ($p < 0.005$). This can be associated with the acidic pH of the beverages, results that are in agreement with previous studies where surface hardness was reduced after immersion in acidic drinks. Considering the results obtained, both null hypotheses were rejected.

The oral cavity is a complex and dynamic environment, and teeth and dental restorations are exposed to a wide range of changes, including thermal or pH changes following consumption of cold, hot, or acidic foods or drinks. Saliva plays also an important role in diluting, neutralizing, and cleaning the oral cavity [32]. Furthermore, beverage and food ingestion are dynamic processes that do not allow for the sustained static retention of fluid in the oral cavity [8]. Therefore, clinical investigations evaluating the real effect of different vegetable juices on colour stability of the aesthetic restorative materials tested in this study may be beneficial. Further investigations may be required to evaluate the effect of different fruit and vegetable juices on colour and mechanical and surface properties of aesthetic restorative materials containing different resin matrices and filler compositions.

In the clinical practice, patients should be aware of the staining effects of the drinks tested in this study, while practitioners should take into consideration the staining susceptibility and the mechanical properties of the resin composites and recommend the ones appropriate to the dietary habits of their patients.

5. Conclusions

Within the limitations of this study, the subsequent conclusions were drawn: Immersion in vegetable juices affected the aesthetic and mechanical properties of the resin composites tested. Colour changes were influenced by the composition of the materials, time of immersion, and vegetable juices. For both resin composites, vegetable juices induced discolouration which increased with exposure time. The highest colour change for Gradia Direct samples was observed after immersion in tomato juice, while Valux Plus samples showed the highest discolouration when immersed in beetroot juice. Change in colour was generally higher in Valux Plus samples compared to Gradia Direct samples, except for samples immersed in tomato juice for seven days. The microhardness of the two materials tested significantly differed due to their compositions. Both resin composites immersed in vegetable juices for seven days showed a lower microhardness than those immersed in distilled water.

Supplementary Materials: The following supporting information can be downloaded at: https://www.mdpi.com/article/10.3390/medicina59040774/s1, Table S1: Colour change ΔE (Mean $\pm$ Standard Error of Mean) for Gradia Direct in different test media at different time points; Table S2: Colour change ΔE (Mean $\pm$ Standard Error of Mean) for Valux Plus samples in different test media at different time points.

Author Contributions: Conceptualization, C.T., E.R.B. and A.N.; formal analysis, C.T., E.R.B. and O.C.I.; investigation, C.T., E.R.B. and C.D.; methodology, C.T., E.R.B., C.D. and A.N.; project administration, C.T., E.R.B. and A.N.; resources, C.T., E.R.B. and A.N.; supervision, A.N.; writing—original draft, C.T.; writing—review & editing, C.T., E.R.B., O.C.I., C.D. and A.N. All authors have read and agreed to the published version of the manuscript.

Funding: This work was supported by the Romania National Council for Higher Education Funding, CNFIS, project number CNFIS-FDI-2022-0259.

Institutional Review Board Statement: Not applicable.

Informed Consent Statement: Not applicable.

Data Availability Statement: All data are available from the corresponding authors.

Conflicts of Interest: The authors declare no conflict of interest.

References

1. Mokeem, L.S.; Garcia, I.M.; Shahkarami, Y.; Blum, L.; Balhaddad, A.A.; Collares, F.M.; Williams, M.A.; Weir, M.D.; Melo, M.A.S. Core-shell nanostructures for improving dental restorative materials: A scoping review of composition, methods, and outcome. *Smart Mater. Med.* **2023**, *4*, 102–110. [CrossRef]
2. Alshehri, A.; Alhalabi, F.; Mustafa, M.; Awad, M.M.; Alqhtani, M.; Almutairi, M.; Alhijab, F.; Jurado, C.A.; Fischer, N.G.; Nurrohman, H.; et al. Effects of Accelerated Aging on Color Stability and Surface Roughness of a Biomimetic Composite: An In Vitro Study. *Biomimetics* **2022**, *7*, 158. [CrossRef] [PubMed]
3. Lai, G.; Zhao, L.; Wang, J.; Kunzelmann, K.H. Surface properties and color stability of dental flowable composites influenced by simulated toothbrushing. *Dent. Mater. J.* **2018**, *37*, 717–724. [CrossRef] [PubMed]
4. Malekipour, M.R.; Sharafi, A.; Kazemi, S.; Khazaei, S.; Shirani, F. Comparison of color stability of a composite resin in different color media. *Dent. Res. J.* **2012**, *9*, 441–446.
5. Veček, N.N.; Par, M.; Sever, E.K.; Miletić, I.; Krmek, S.J. The Effect of a Green Smoothie on Microhardness, Profile Roughness and Color Change of Dental Restorative Materials. *Polymers* **2022**, *14*, 2067. [CrossRef]
6. Borges, M.G.; Soares, C.J.; Maia, T.S.; Bicalho, A.A.; Barbosa, T.P.; Costa, H.L.; Menezes, M.S. Effect of Acidic Drinks on Shade Matching, Surface Topography, and Mechanical Properties of Conventional and Bulk-Fill Composite Resins. *J. Prosthet. Dent.* **2019**, *121*, 868.e1–868.e8. [CrossRef]
7. Choi, J.W.; Lee, M.J.; Oh, S.H.; Kim, K.-M. Changes in the Physical Properties and Color Stability of Aesthetic Restorative Materials Caused by Various Beverages. *Dent. Mater. J.* **2019**, *38*, 33–40. [CrossRef]
8. Ren, Y.F.; Lin Feng, L.; Serban, D.; Malmstrom, H.S. Effects of common beverage colorants on color stability of dental composite resins: The utility of a thermocycling stain challenge model in vitro. *J. Dent.* **2012**, *40*, 48–56. [CrossRef]
9. Meshki, R.; Rashidi, M. Effect of natural and commercially produced juices on colour stability of microhybrid and nanohybrid composites. *BDJ Open* **2022**, *8*, 1. [CrossRef]
10. Faris, T.M.; Abdulrahim, R.H.; Mahmood, M.A.; Dalloo, G.A.M.; Gul, S.S. In vitro evaluation of dental color stability using various aesthetic restorative materials after immersion in different drinks. *BMC Oral Health* **2023**, *23*, 49. [CrossRef]
11. Gawriołek, M.; Gawriołek, K.; Eliasz, W.; Czarnecka, B.; Paszynska, E.; Sikorski, M. How Does the Color of Restorative Material Change during Exposure to Dietary Liquids Due to the Acquisition of a Discolored Layer? *Coatings* **2020**, *10*, 866. [CrossRef]
12. Manojlovic, D.; Lenhardt, L.; Milićević, B.; Antonov, M.; Miletic, V.; Dramićanin, M.D. Evaluation of Staining-Dependent Colour Changes in Resin Composites Using Principal Component Analysis. *Sci. Rep.* **2015**, *5*, 14638. [CrossRef]
13. Sakineh, N.; Abbas, A.; Mohsen, P. Effects of beverage colorants and accelerated aging on the color stability of indirect resin composites. *J. Dent. Sci.* **2012**, *7*, 231–237. [CrossRef]
14. Tanthanuch, S.; Kukiattrakoon, B.; Eiam-O-Pas, K.; Pokawattana, K.; Pamanee, N.; Thongkamkaew, W.; Kochatung, A. Surface changes of various bulk-fill resin-based composites after exposure to different food-simulating liquid and beverages. *J. Esthet. Restor. Dent.* **2018**, *30*, 126–135. [CrossRef] [PubMed]
15. Al-Haj Ali, S.N.; Alsulaim, H.N.; Albarrak, M.I.; Farah, R.I. Spectrophotometric comparison of color stability of microhybrid and nanocomposites following exposure to common soft drinks among adolescents: An in vitro study. *Eur. Arch. Paediatr. Dent.* **2021**, *22*, 675–683. [CrossRef] [PubMed]
16. Al Kheraif, A.A.; Qasim, S.S.; Ramakrishnaiah, R.; Rehman, I.U. Effect of different beverages on the color stability and degree of conversion of nano and microhybrid composites. *Dent. Mater. J.* **2013**, *32*, 326–331. [CrossRef] [PubMed]
17. Bansal, K.; Acharya, S.R.; Saraswathi, V. Effect of alcoholic and non-alcoholic beverages on colour stability and surface roughness of resin composites: An in vitro study. *J. Conserv. Dent.* **2012**, *15*, 283–288. [CrossRef] [PubMed]
18. Raczyk, M.; Kruszewski, B.; Zachariasz, E. Effect of Tomato, Beetroot and Carrot Juice Addition on Physicochemical, Antioxidant and Texture Properties of Wheat Bread. *Antioxidants* **2022**, *11*, 2178. [CrossRef] [PubMed]
19. Al-Qarni, M.A.; Das, G.; Saquib, S.; Sibghatullah, M.; Alahmari, M.M.; Arora, S. The Effect of Arabian Coffee, Black Tea and Orange-juice on Microhardness and Color Stability of Hybrid Composite Resins. An in vitro Study. *Mater. Plast.* **2021**, *58*, 218–22. [CrossRef]
20. Available online: https://www.gc.dental/europe/sites/europe.gc.dental/files/products/downloads/gradiadirectloflo/sds_SDS_Gradia_Direct_LoFlo_EU.pdf (accessed on 20 January 2023).
21. Available online: https://multimedia.3m.com/mws/mediawebserver?SSSSSuUn_zu8l00xl8_1m821nv70k17zHvu9lxtD7SSSSSS-- (accessed on 20 January 2023).
22. Danesh, K.A.; Johar, N. Comparison of Different Bleaching Treatments Effect on Micro Hardness of Four Different Aged Composites. *Jentashapir. J. Cell Mol. Biol.* **2016**, *7*, 39039. [CrossRef]
23. Kocaagaoglu, H.; Aslan, T.; Gürbulak, A.; Albayrak, H.; Taşdemir, Z.; Gumus, H. Efficacy of polishing kits on the surface roughness and color stability of different composite resins. *Niger J. Clin. Pract.* **2017**, *20*, 557–565. [CrossRef]

24. Yap, A.U.; Mah, M.K.; Lye, C.P.; Loh, P.L. Influence of dietary simulating solvents on the hardness of provisional restorative materials. *Dental. Mater.* **2004**, *20*, 370–376. [CrossRef]
25. Li, Y.; Swartz, M.L.; Phillips, R.W.; Moore, B.K.; Roberts, T.A. Materials Science Effect of Filler Content and Size on Properties of Composites. *J. Dent. Res.* **1985**, *64*, 1396–1403. [CrossRef] [PubMed]
26. Kim, K.H.; Ong, J.L.; Okuno, O. The effect of filler loading and morphology on the mechanical properties of contemporary composites. *J. Prosthet. Dent.* **2002**, *87*, 642–649. [CrossRef]
27. Yew, H.; Berekally, T.; Richards, L. A laboratory investigation of colour changes in two contemporary resin composites on exposure to spices. *Aust. Dent. J.* **2013**, *58*, 468–477. [CrossRef]
28. Wongkhantee, S.; Patanapiradej, V.; Maneenut, C.; Tantbirojn, D. Effect of acidic food and drinks on surface hardness of enamel, dentine, and tooth-coloured filling materials. *J. Dent.* **2006**, *34*, 214–220. [CrossRef]
29. Gupta, R.; Madan, M.; Dua, P.; Saini, S.; Mangla, R.; Kainthla, T.; Dupper, A. Comparative Evaluation of Microhardness by Common Drinks on Esthetic Restorative Materials and Enamel: An in vitro Study. *Int. J. Clin. Pediatr. Dent.* **2018**, *11*, 155–160. [CrossRef] [PubMed]
30. Poggio, C.; Viola, M.; Mirando, M.; Chiesa, M.; Beltrami, R.; Colombo, M. Microhardness of different esthetic restorative materials: Evaluation and comparison after exposure to acidic drink. *Dent. Res. J.* **2018**, *15*, 166–172. [CrossRef]
31. Hengtrakool, C.; Kukiattrakoon, B.; Kedjarune-Leggat, U. Effect of naturally acidic agents on microhardness and surface micromorphology of restorative materials. *Eur. J. Dent.* **2011**, *5*, 89–100. [CrossRef] [PubMed]
32. Cunha-Cruz, J.; Scott, J.; Rothen, M.; Mancl, L.; Lawhorn, T.; Brossel, K.; Berg, J. Northwest Practice-based Research Collaborative in Evidence-based Dentistry. Salivary characteristics and dental caries: Evidence from general dental practices. *J. Am. Dent. Assoc.* **2013**, *144*, 31–40. [CrossRef]

Disclaimer/Publisher's Note: The statements, opinions and data contained in all publications are solely those of the individual author(s) and contributor(s) and not of MDPI and/or the editor(s). MDPI and/or the editor(s) disclaim responsibility for any injury to people or property resulting from any ideas, methods, instructions or products referred to in the content.

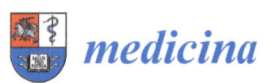

Case Report

Introducing an Innovative Approach for Managing Proximal Non-Cavitated Carious Lesions in Juvenile Permanent Dentition: Combining Orthodontic Separators and Silver Fluoride Application

Eilaf E. A. Ahmed, Salma Al Nesser and Julian Schmoeckel *

Department Preventive and Pediatric Dentistry, University Medicine Greifswald, Walther-Rathenau Straße 42a, 17487 Greifswald, Germany; eilafeltigani@gmail.com (E.E.A.A.); salma.alnesser93@gmail.com (S.A.N.)
* Correspondence: julian.schmoeckel@uni-greifswald.de

Citation: Ahmed, E.E.A.; Al Nesser, S.; Schmoeckel, J. Introducing an Innovative Approach for Managing Proximal Non-Cavitated Carious Lesions in Juvenile Permanent Dentition: Combining Orthodontic Separators and Silver Fluoride Application. *Medicina* **2023**, *59*, 1892. https://doi.org/10.3390/medicina59111892

Academic Editors: Yanfang Ren and Vita Maciulskiene

Received: 20 September 2023
Revised: 14 October 2023
Accepted: 20 October 2023
Published: 25 October 2023

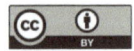

Copyright: © 2023 by the authors. Licensee MDPI, Basel, Switzerland. This article is an open access article distributed under the terms and conditions of the Creative Commons Attribution (CC BY) license (https://creativecommons.org/licenses/by/4.0/).

Abstract: Background and Objectives: The aim was to introduce an innovative, easy and cheap clinical approach for the control of multiple proximal non-cavitated lesions via the application of 38% silver fluoride after placement of orthodontic separators in the permanent dentition in high-caries-risk children. Materials and Methods: The case series describes the management of initial proximal carious lesions using silver fluoride (SF) products in the permanent dentition of two adolescent patients with prior proximal caries progression. Both presented with multiple asymptomatic carious lesions that were identified through the use of bitewing radiographs and classified according to the ADA proximal caries classification system. Using orthodontic separators prior to the planned application of SF, most of the surfaces could then be quickly directly examined to check for surface integrity. Follow-up examinations were conducted clinically and radiographically for at least one year to monitor lesion progression. Results: None of the 25 enamel lesions (E1/E2) exhibited signs of progression after single SF application, while 2 out of 11 dentine lesions (D1) showed progression and required restorative intervention. The progressed lesions potentially had non-cleansable micro-cavitations that were either clinically undetected or not fully reached with the micro-brush in SF application. Thus, this should have been repeated or combined with SF application via soaked superfloss to potentially achieve better results. Conclusions: Single application of 38% silver fluoride directly onto active enamel lesions in juvenile permanent teeth with the prior use of orthodontic separators combined with a caries-risk-specific prevention program appears to be highly effective and should be considered as a viable minimally invasive option for patients and clinicians due to its cost-effectiveness and time efficiency.

Keywords: initial caries; silver fluoride; minimal invasive; caries diagnosis

1. Introduction

Dental caries are dynamic, with an imbalance between remineralization and demineralization of the dental surface [1], and initial lesions are the earliest stage of this process. These develop when the enamel is demineralized under the subsurface beneath an intact surface layer of enamel [2]. These initial lesions can be reversed or arrested if remineralization outweighs the demineralization process, or transformed into a cavitation if demineralization outweighs the remineralization process [3].

Active initial caries appear clinically as chalky white lesions [4] and can be easily diagnosed on cleaned and dried occlusal or smooth surfaces. On the contrary, proximal surfaces have always been a challenge regarding the early diagnosis and consequently the control and management of the caries process. Clinical diagnosis within the area of contact points, limited salivary access and the inability to self-cleanse have shaped this challenge. In general, the caries process in the proximal area of the permanent dentition in low-caries-risk children is slow, especially in countries where a significant caries decline in children has been observed [5]. Nonetheless, caries incidence during adolescence is still high and mainly affects proximal surfaces.

Management of such lesions can range from improving oral hygiene practices and fluoride use to the application of proximal sealants, caries infiltration and traditional restorations [6]. Silver fluoride products (SF) offer a minimally invasive treatment option that has been shown to be effective in managing carious lesions in children and adults [7].

In addition to the gold-standard X-rays, alternative methods have been introduced over the last few decades for detecting caries without the use of radiation, such as optical coherence tomography (OCT) and near-infrared (NIR) and fiber-optic technology, which have contributed to the recently developed digital fiber optics (FOTI/DIFOTI) [8,9]. Using these methods together enables early diagnosis, potentially shifting the intervention from surgical to preventive treatment [3].

It is quite well known that SF provides significant chemical interference in the progression of caries and also has the ability to prevent the initiation of the caries process [10] for both primary and permanent teeth [11,12]. It has been recommended from in vitro studies that, especially in non-compliant patients, 38% SF be applied to remineralize incipient caries lesions of permanent teeth where aesthetics is not a concern [13], as it is capable of inducing/increasing enamel remineralization [7,14].

To the best of our knowledge, no clinical studies or case reports are available in the literature on SF treatment of multiple active non-cavitated proximal carious lesions in permanent dentition of children, despite the demonstrated high effectiveness of SF for all stages of carious lesions.

This case series was prepared following the CARE Guidelines [15], and aims to introduce an innovative, easy and cheap clinical approach for the control of multiple proximal non-cavitated lesions via the application of 38% silver fluoride after placement of orthodontic separators for direct clinical inspection and better access to the proximal lesion.

2. Case Presentations

Case 1

Patient information

In November 2019, a 13-year-old female patient in good health visited the Department of Preventive and Pediatric Dentistry at the University of Greifswald for a routine dental check-up, accompanied by her parents.

Clinical findings

The patient did not report any symptoms or complaints. During the dental examination, poor oral hygiene and a history of consuming sugary foods and drinks were documented. Dental history revealed that the patient had worn a fixed orthodontic appliance for 18 months, which might have negatively affected the patient's oral hygiene and caries activity. The clinical examination (11/2019) revealed a suspicion of multiple proximal carious lesions.

Diagnostic assessments

1. **Clinical diagnostics:** Proximal surfaces were screened with a near-infrared imaging system and revealed the presence of both enamel and dentine lesions.
2. **Bitewings radiographs:** During the same dental visit, bitewing X-rays were taken to confirm the presence of lesions and to determine their depth and proximity to the pulp (Figure 1). The ADA proximal caries classification system was used to diagnose and monitor progression of these lesions: E1: lesion in the outer half of the enamel; E2: lesion within the inner half of the enamel; D1: lesion passing the enamel dentin junction (EDJ) and within the outer third of dentin; D2: lesion within the 2nd third of the dentine; D3: deep lesion passing the 2nd third of the dentin [16]. For evaluations of the bitewing X-rays, three calibrated pediatric dentists classified the lesions independently in a dark room with the option to digitally modify the contrast and brightness of the X-rays. In the rare cases of disagreement, consent was reached

via a discussion (Table 1). Bitewings were taken using a Sirona Heliodent DS and a Xios XG supreme intraoral sensor, with a standard dose of 0.16 mAs. The same criteria for bitewings were considered also for the follow-up visit which was at the same time the pre-SDF radiographic examination (Figure 2).

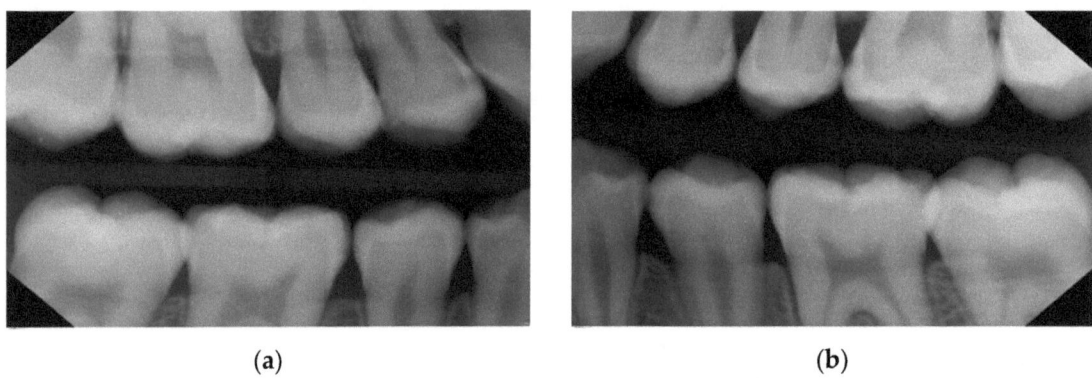

(a)   (b)

Figure 1. Case 1—Baseline in 11/2019: Bitewings show multiple proximal lesions but without clear cavitation on the right (**a**) and left side (**b**). The patient was 13 years old and had a history of fixed orthodontic appliances. Only non-invasive caries management options were undertaken, as due to COVID-19 pandemic, the patient did not show up for micro-invasive or restorative treatment until 2022—see Figure 2. For a Lesion assessment, see Table 1.

Table 1. Stages of carious lesions radiographically for case 1 at baseline 11/2019 (pre-pandemic); in 02/2022 (before SF application and restorative treatment); and 1.5 years later in 06/2023 as follow-up after the SF application in both upper and lower permanent teeth for this highly caries active adolescent patient, documented by caries progression in the first years (from 2019 to 2022) and stability from after SF application and restorative treatment (from 2022 to 2023).

Tooth	17		16		15		14		24		25		26		27
Surface	M	D	M	D	M	D	M	D	M	D	M	D	M	D	M
Figure 1—11/2019	?	0	E1	E2	E2	E2	D1		0	D1	E2	D1	D2	0	0
Figure 2—02/2022	?	D1	D1	D1	E2	D1	-		-	D2	D1	D1	D3	E2	?
Figure 6—07/2023	?	D1	D1	D1	E2	D1	F		0	F	F	D1	F	E2	0

Tooth	47		46		45		44		34		35		36		37
Surface	M	D	M	D	M	D	M	D	D		M	D	M	D	M
Figure 1—11/2019	0	0	E1	E1	0	0			E2		E1	E2	0	0	?
Figure 2—02/2022	0	0	E1	E2	0	0			E2		E1	E2	E1	E1	?
Figure 6—07/2023	0	0	E1	E2	0	0			E2		E1	E2	E1	?	0

(?) = cannot be assessed, (-) = not included in the X-ray, (F) = filling.

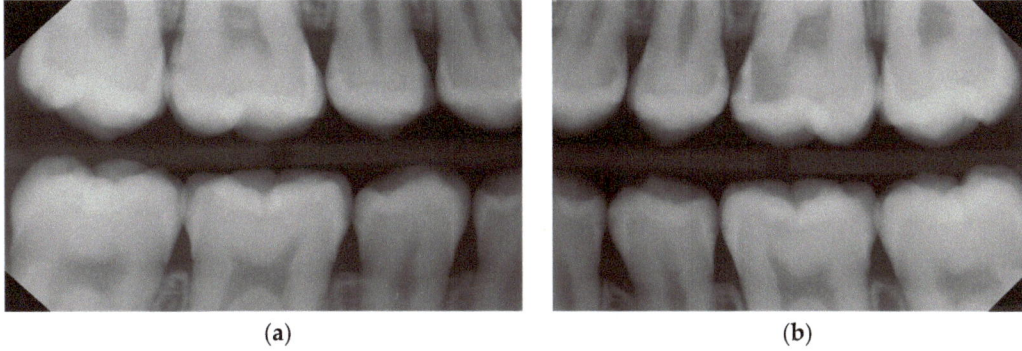

Figure 2. Case 1—After more than 2 years, the bitewings on the right (**a**) and left side (**b**) in 02/2022 show caries progression with a solely non-invasive caries management approach, like instructions to floss and apply fluoride varnish, before the COVID-19 pandemic. The patient is now 15 years old, and the bitewings depict the status before the decision to apply SF on the initial/non-cavitated lesions alongside the restorative treatment (composite restorations in moderate lesions, and for the deep lesion in tooth 26, selective caries removal with the application of biodentine (Septodont) prior to the restoration); see Figure 3; for a lesion assessment, see Table 1.

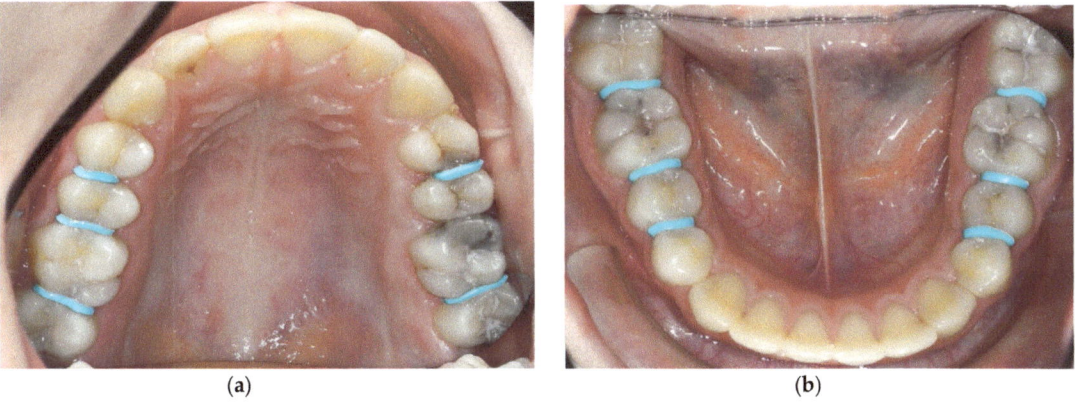

Figure 3. Clinical photos after placement of orthodontic separators proximally but prior to SF application (04/2022, patient's age: 15 years) in the upper (**a**) and lower jaw (**b**). Tooth 26 was already treated restoratively occluso-mesially with selective caries removal and indirect pulp capping with biodentine. The black staining in 26 occurred due to SF application on the distal lesion of 25 after tooth preparation and biodentine application but before composite filling in 26, as the D1 lesion in 25 was distally clinically non-cavitated (similar to 24).

3. **Tooth separation with orthodontic rubbers:** This revealed the absence of cavitation (Figure 3a,b).

These methods were used together as it was found that a combination of all three methods could improve the number of carious lesions detected [17].

In total, 15 initial (non-cavitated) lesions were detected radiographically (02/2022): 9 enamel lesions (E1, E2) and 6 (D1) dentine lesions (Figure 2). Moreover, the high plaque and gingival bleeding index of the patient indicated that the proximal lesions were very likely active [16,18].

Therapeutic intervention

1. **Prophylaxis program**

Within the preventive concept in the department, during the same visit, a non-operative approach was taken to control the initial caries lesions. This approach included providing the patient with oral hygiene instructions, diet counselling, dental floss instructions and fluoride varnish every three months to arrest the progression of the lesions, as she was considered to be a high-caries-risk patient.

A disclosing solution was used to show the dental plaque for both the child and their parents. Then, the child was asked to brush their teeth alone with the use of a normal toothbrush with a fluoridated toothpaste to see if this child was brushing his teeth correctly. After that, the child had their teeth cleaned by the dentist using an electric toothbrush attached to a low-speed handpiece. Unfortunately, this was not sufficient, as indicated by the following clinical and radiographical examinations. Likely due to the COVID-19 pandemic and its restrictions, the patient neither followed the recommendations of regular follow-up nor of micro-invasive and/or restorative approaches, for instance, for the teeth 14, 24 and 26.

2. **Indicated use of SF**

After a long time span of 27 months from the first bitewings (11/2019), new bitewing X-rays were taken (02/2022), which revealed, in line with the clinical findings, a clear progression of the existing proximal lesions and development of new lesions. This highlights the caries activity of the patient (Figure 2). The stage and location of the proximal lesions are listed in detail (Table 1). Micro-invasive treatment options such as resin infiltration were recommended for management of the non-cavitated lesions (E1, E2, D1) and restoration of the moderate to deep lesions. In contrast to the first visit, the use of silver fluoride products had tremendously increased in the department due to the COVID-19 pandemic. Therefore, this time, the novel "experimental" application method with SF presented in this article was also offered. The patient and parents were provided with a detailed explanation of the treatment options, including their advantages, disadvantages, time and cost. Following the discussion, it was agreed to apply SF (riva star, SDI) to all proximal areas with initial proximal lesions. Composite restorations were planned for moderate lesions, and for the deep lesion in tooth 26, selective caries removal with the application of biodentine (Septodont) prior the restoration was performed, and silver fluoride was applied directly on the distal surface of 25 in case no cavitation was present during the restorative session for tooth 26.

Treatment steps of for managing active initial/likely non-cavitated proximal caries lesions

(1) **Placement of orthodontic separators**

Separators were placed in all approximal areas with initial proximal caries lesions for two hours to facilitate direct clinical inspection and direct application of SF using a micro-brush (Figure 3). After removing the separators, a short time span of approximately 5–10 s was used for direct clinical examination. Then, SF was applied quickly with a small micro-brush was used in the proximal areas (Figure 4). It is important to note that the proximal contact area was not always fully open to allow complete insertion of the micro-brush in all surfaces over the entire application time. Still, the prior tooth separation improved accessibility for an initial short clinical examination and facilitated the flow of the SF to the lesion. In case of a clear sign of a manifest cavitation, restoration would have been planned.

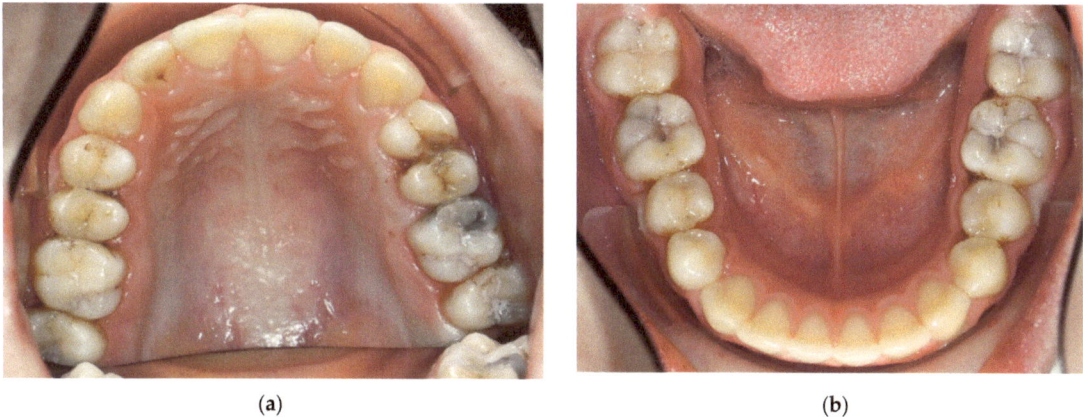

(a)   (b)

Figure 4. Clinical photos in 04/2022 directly after application of SF (riva star, SDI) in upper (**a**) and lower jaw (**b**); same day as application of separators for 2 h; patient's age: 15 years. Partial irritation and black staining of the gums can be seen interproximally, which usually disappears within a few days and does not cause long-term effects as the follow-up photos (see Figure 5) demonstrate.

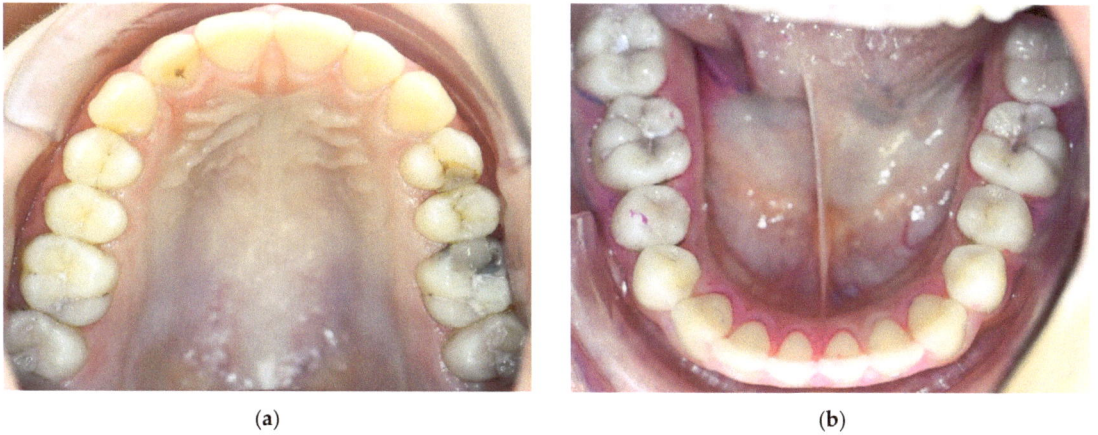

(a)   (b)

Figure 5. One-year follow-up after SF in 06/2023; patient's age: 17 years. Clinical photos after staining the plaque and self-brushing of the patient. Composite restorations on 24 and 26 unfortunately still show the discolorations due to SF application on neighboring teeth during the same treatment session (**a**). The staining of the other initial proximal lesions is not or is barely visible and does not cause aesthetic concerns (**b**). Possibly a re-application of SF to the proximal lesions should be considered.

(2)   **SF application (Riva Star®, SDI)**

- Petroleum gel was used to protect and avoid/reduce staining of lips and surrounding extra-oral soft tissue [19].
- Other tooth surfaces were isolated using cotton rolls and a saliva ejector to minimize unwanted staining or irritation of soft tissue or other surfaces.
- Using air, the area was dried before application of the material.
- SF was applied using a micro-brush for about 30 s to one minute per proximal area [20].
- A light curing of 10 s for each proximal space was used to accelerate activation of SF and to allow SF to penetrate deeper into the lesion [21].

- Fluoride varnish (Duraphat, 22.600 ppm) was applied on top of the area to keep the SF in contact with the caries lesion or high-risk surface for as long as possible to prevent saliva from diluting the SF, and most importantly to mask the ammonia taste from the SF product [22,23].

Follow-up for re-evaluation of the single-time SF application

The patient was followed up clinically every 4 to 6 months using the standard prophylaxis program (Figure 5). After 16 months from the last bitewing, another bitewing was planned to assess the progression of the existing lesions and the development of new lesions. The radiographs revealed that there was no evidence of development of new caries lesions. All enamel lesions were stable and did not show signs of caries progression. Among the D1 lesions, one out of six lesions showed signs of cavitation clinically, and required restoration. None of the other dentin lesions displayed radiographic evidence of caries progression (Figure 6 and Table 2).

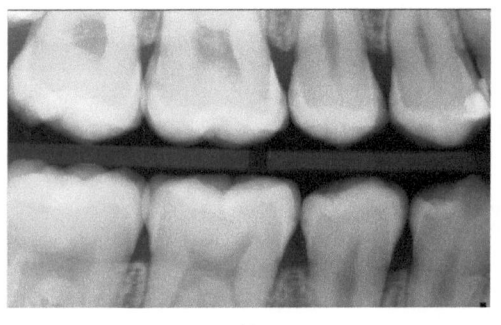 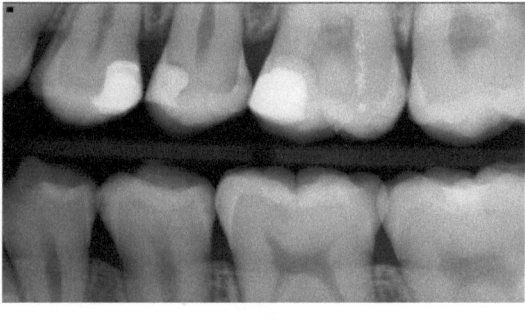

(a) (b)

Figure 6. Bitewings on the right (a) and left side (b) 16 months after SF application show the stages of proximal lesions as well as the integrity of the restorative procedures (06/2023, age: 17 years old) indicating a clear reduction in caries activity and stability of the lesions. For a lesions assessment, see Table 1.

Table 2. Case 2: Stages of the carious lesions radiographically at baseline in 2019 in the upper jaw and lower jaw, just before SF application in 2022 and 1 year later in 2023 in both upper and lower permanent teeth for this highly caries active adolescent patient documented by the caries progression from 2019 to 2022.

Tooth	17		16		15		14		24		25		26		27
Surface	M	D	M	D	M	D	M	M	D	M	D	M	D	M
Figure 7—02/2019	0	0	E1	0	0	0	0	0	0	0	E1	D1	0	0
Figure 8—03/2022	E1	D1	E1	E2	D1	E2	0	0	D2	D1	D1	D2	E1	E1
Figure 10—03/2023	E1	D1	E1	E2	D1	E2	0	0	D2	D1	D3	D2	E1	0
Tooth	47		46		45		44		34		35		36		37
Surface	M	D	M	D	M	D	M	D	D	M	D	M	D	M
Figure 7—02/2019	0	0	0	0	0	0	0	0	0	0	0	0	E1	0
Figure 8—03/2022	E1	D1	E1	E1	E2	E1	E1	E2	E1	E1	D2	E1
Figure 10—03/2023	E1	D1	E1	E1	E2	E1	E1	E2	E1	E1	F	E1

(?)= cannot be assessed, (-) = not included on the X-ray, (F) = filling.

Case 2
Patient information

A 13-year-old male patient had been attending the clinic for dental check-ups for approximately seven years. The patient had a medical history of neurodermatitis. His dental history indicated a poor oral hygiene, an uncontrolled diet, and high caries experience in primary molars, most of which were treated in the department to which he was initially referred due to his low cooperative behavior with the family dentist.

Clinical findings

The patient's average proximal plaque index was ~60%, and the gingival bleeding index was ~30%. Despite receiving instructions to improve his oral hygiene and diet, including the recommendation to use fluoride gel (12,600 ppm) once a week at home and dental floss (although it was likely not consistently used), the presence of smooth surface initial caries and a high-caries-risk for the patient remained evident.

Diagnostic assessments

Diagnosis was made using the same diagnostic tools as in the first patient. Bitewing reading showed multiple initial caries lesions on posterior teeth but no clearly cavitated proximal lesion (Figure 7 and Table 2). In total, 21 initial proximal lesions were detected: 16 enamel lesions (E1, E2) and 5 dentine lesions (D1). The lesions were more likely to be active according to the high plaque and gingival bleeding index.

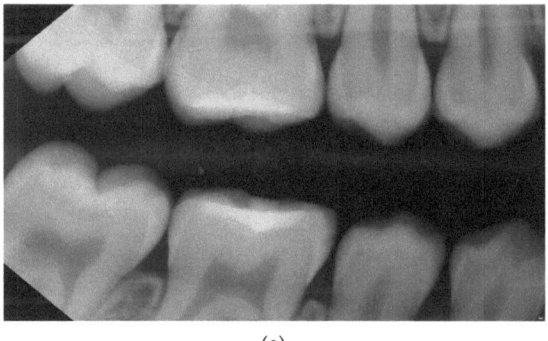 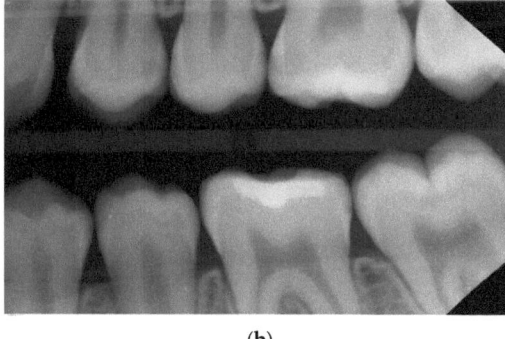

(a) (b)

Figure 7. Case 2—Baseline: bitewings in 2019 show the proximal non-cavitated lesions on the right (**a**) and the left side (**b**) at the age of 13. Only non-invasive caries management options including regular recall and fluoride varnish application were undertaken at this point. For a lesion assessment, see Table 2.

Therapeutic intervention

1. Prophylaxis program

The patient was given instructions on oral hygiene and the use of dental floss regularly, in addition to the prophylaxis program at the dental department, which was the same as for the first patient. The patient was scheduled for application of fluoride varnish every 3–4 months. In contrast to case report one, this patient attended all of his appointments regularly, except for only one missed appointment during the COVID-19 pandemic lockdown. Despite regular appointments and instructions, the patient's oral hygiene had barely improved and the sugary drinks were still consumed on a regular basis.

Indicated use of SF and treatment steps

After approximately three years from the first bitewings, new bitewings were taken, which revealed the presence of new caries lesions and progression of the previous proximal lesions, showing that the high caries risk recall program was not sufficient (Figure 8). The stages and locations of the initial proximal lesions are listed in detail (Table 2). After discussing the various alternatives with the parents and the child, taking into account the cost, time and feasibility, it was decided to use SF for all initial lesions and composite fillings for moderate lesions with cavitation (which are paid for by health insurance within the German reimbursement system until the age of 15). For D1 lesions, as they were clinically not detectable at all, it was agreed to place separators for a better assessment of surface integrity (Figure 9a,b). The patient was to be followed up regularly, and if cavitation was present, fillings would be performed. Separators and SDF were applied to a total of 19 initial lesions using the same procedure as in the first patient (Figure 9a,b), and the patient was scheduled for follow-up about every 3 months with fluoride varnish application. The clinical photos show, in addition to what was depicted in case one, that sometimes not all separators remained in their spot even after only two hours (Figure 9a,b). Unfortunately, the more separators are applied in one quadrant, the less space is gained proximally and the less time there is to investigate the proximal surfaces and apply the SF. Furthermore, this illustrates the black staining on the healthy enamel after SF application and light curing. This staining will disappear with brushing at home or can also be brushed away with a polishing paste in the office (Figure 9c,d).

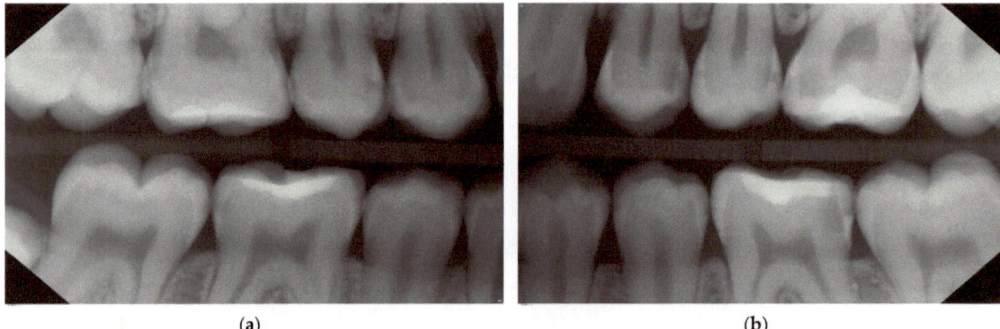

Figure 8. Case 2—Bitewings on the right (**a**) and left side (**b**) after slightly more than three years in 2022 show the progression and development of new proximal caries lesions. At this stage, at the age of almost 16, the decision was taken to apply SF proximally; 36 was treated with a composite restoration due to a clinically assessed cavitation. For a lesion assessment, see Table 2.

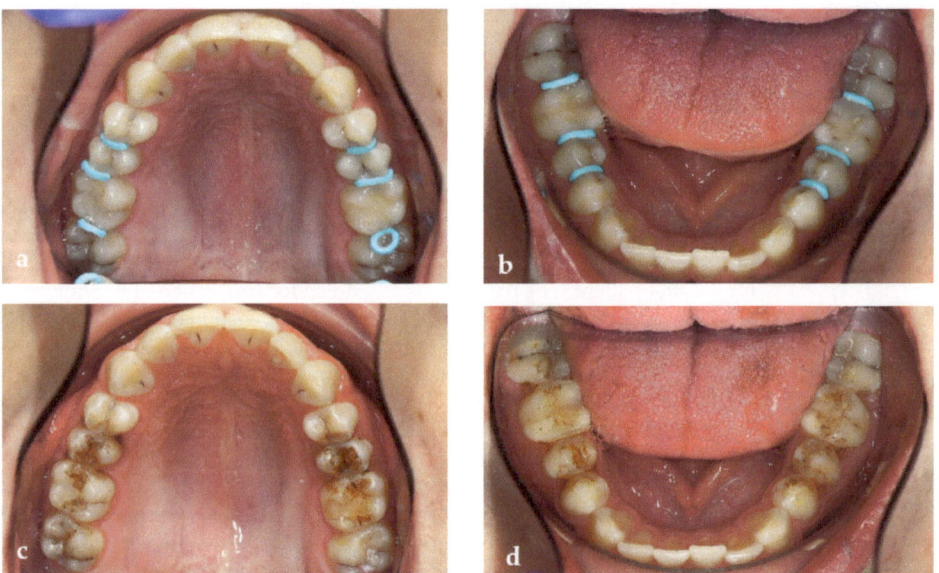

Figure 9. Clinical photos in 2022 (patient's age is almost 16) after applying the orthodontic separators proximally in the upper (**a**) and lower jaw (**b**) and immediately after SF application and light curing (**c,d**). The black staining on the healthy enamel will disappear with brushing at home or can also be brushed away with a polishing paste in the office.

Follow-up for re-evaluation of SF

In March 2023, one year after the last bitewing, new bitewing radiographs were taken to assess the progression of the existing lesions, with a specific focus on the D1 lesions. The radiographs revealed that there was no evidence for development of new caries lesions. All enamel lesions were stable and did not show signs of caries progression. Among D1 lesions, only one out of five lesions showed caries progression regarding the classification system (Table 2), but some other dentine lesions progressed slightly within their category (e.g., D1 or D2) and restorative measures were planned (Figure 10). Interestingly, caries progression was only observed in the second quadrant, so despite the tooth separation, micro-cavitation possibly remained undetected due to the short examination time or due to the fact that SF could not be sufficiently applied to these lesions.

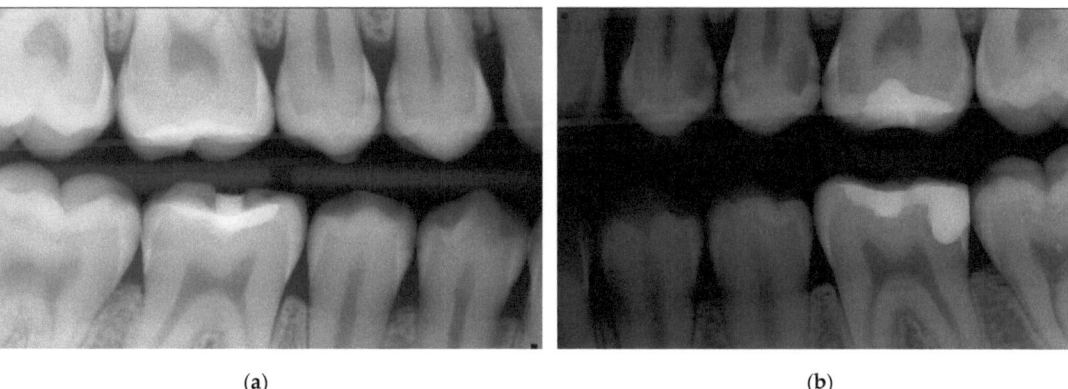

(a) (b)

Figure 10. Case 2—Bitewings (03/2023) on the right (**a**) and left side (**b**) at the 1-year follow-up after SF application. The patient's age is almost 17. The radiographic situation shows both the progression (only in second quadrant (**b**)) and stagnation of (both enamel and D1) proximal lesions after single application of SF within regular recall visits.

3. Discussion

The main focus in managing initial caries lesions should be on non-operative treatment, aiming to avoid or delay restorative measures by enhancing remineralization to arrest lesion progression, or at best, reverse it. Though it is well evident that approximal initial caries can be treated non-operatively, as lesions confined to the EDJ are most likely non-cavitated (only 8–19% are cavitated), most dentists tend to intervene surgically in such lesions in permanent teeth. This could be concerning, as dental restorations have a limited lifespan; thus, initiating a restorative cycle will eventually compromise the integrity and survival of the tooth [24–26].

To best implement minimal intervention measures, early diagnosis is the primary objective [27]. Conventional bitewings remain the gold standard to diagnose and detect approximal lesions, though they have a low sensitivity for the detection of early lesions extending only to the outer enamel, this ranges from 51 to 64% for enamel lesions and is 67% for caries reaching the enamel–dentin junction (EDJ) [28,29]. This means that 33% of lesions confined to the EDJ may go undiagnosed. The sensitivity is probably even lower in real-world settings, where the quality of the radiographs is not always optimal. To enhance the standardization of lesion monitoring and ensure consistent radiation direction, the utilization of individualized bitewing holders would be a valuable additional tool. Therefore, it is advisable to use bitewings in conjunction with other diagnostic tools (as, e.g., tooth separation for direct clinical examination, NIR or FOTI) for a comprehensive assessment.

Nonetheless, in the context of monitoring lesions, bitewing radiography offers a suitable sensitivity and specificity for early detection without a significantly increased risk of false positives. Moreover, bitewings become increasingly sensitive as lesions progress, which enhances their effectiveness in assessing progressed lesions compared to their initial baseline assessment. Still, irrespective of the treatment performed, dentists should be cautious in diagnosing non-progression from enamel to EDJ lesions, as a certain risk of underestimation remains due to the described diagnostic limitations.

In Germany, this is typically recommended to be performed at intervals determined by the patient's caries risk. Bitewings in high-risk children should be considered about every 12–24 months [30].

SF has been proven to be highly effective in preventing caries development and arresting ~80% of dentine carious lesions in high-caries risk patients [31,32]. Moreover, unlike other micro-invasive techniques, which create a mechanical barrier against the biofilm [33], SF works in a biological way, as the distinctive anti-microbial activity and high fluoride content not only arrest caries, but also promote remineralization [21]. This has been demonstrated in retrospective and in vitro studies [34].

This case series demonstrated that SF was highly effective in preventing the progression of enamel carious lesions (E1 and E2), as no evidence of progression was observed even in highly caries active adolescents. However, SF was less effective in dentin lesions (D1), with still only two out of eleven lesions showing progression and requiring restorative treatment. The reduced efficacy of SF in D1 lesions may be attributed to a higher bacterial load and deeper bacterial penetration into the dentin. These micro-cavitations are difficult to clean, can protect the biofilm and consequently facilitate the progression of caries [30,35]. This could be due to an incorrect clinical baseline assessment (cavitation not seen), insufficient use of the micro-brush to apply the SF or persisting caries activity in the patient due to, e.g., irregular home use of dental floss, insufficient fluoride uses and/or a high frequency of sugar intake.

In line with the existing literature, these cases show that non-invasive approaches, including fluoridated toothpaste, flossing and fluoride products, proved insufficient to arrest caries progression or to prevent its development in high-caries-risk patients. Although dental flossing is a suitable method for mechanical plaque removal from proximal surfaces [36,37], it is not widely practiced among the general population [9]. Therefore, the effectiveness of this approach relies largely on patient compliance, which may lead to an insufficient level of lesion management [38–40].

Micro-invasive approaches, such as proximal sealants and resin infiltration, demonstrate a high amount of evidence in reducing the risk of caries progression. However, they are time-consuming and more expensive. For instance, the time required to place proximal sealants or infiltrants is roughly comparable to the time required for a two-surface composite filling. Moreover, these treatment options are technique-sensitive for both patients and operators [41–43]. This complexity is further compounded when multiple surfaces are involved.

SF application was demonstrated to be easy, simple, quick and time-efficient in the sense that it allows for the management of multiple surfaces at a time. Despite involving a two-visit dental procedure, the procedural time on the dental chair is relatively short, especially when compared to treatment alternatives (e.g., caries infiltration) for a high number of lesions. Additionally, the use of SF-soaked superfloss could always be considered to eliminate the need for an additional appointment for separator placement when not feasible, but this comes with the drawback of lacking direct clinical assessment. Furthermore, SF is highly cost-efficient, accessible and equitable for all socio-economic groups, making it a valuable option not only in Europe but also worldwide.

Caries arrest using SF is considered a safe treatment, and it rarely causes any local symptoms such as pain or gum swelling [44]. The only apparent drawback of SF is the dark staining of the lesions, and acceptance of the staining varies with different cultures and the affected teeth or surface. However, in general, the acceptance of the staining in posterior teeth is far better than in anterior teeth [45]. More importantly, as demonstrated in this case series, black staining of the (arrested) proximal lesions caused by SF was hardly visible due to the tight contact surfaces of permanent teeth (Figures 4 and 5), but staining of composite fillings may occur when applied in the same session before the restoration itself.

We want to highlight that this approach is highly innovative and has not been reported in the literature. It has demonstrated high effectiveness for managing initial enamel proximal lesions. However, for dentine lesions, it may be advisable to consider multiple applications, possibly in the 3- or 6-month follow-up visits.

We strongly emphasize the importance of conducting different types of clinical research in this area to establish evidence for the effectiveness of SF application in managing initial proximal carious lesions using various techniques, preferably RCTs comparing the efficacy of SF with, e.g., other fluoride varnishes, caries infiltration or self-assembling peptides, should be taken into consideration.

4. Conclusions

The application of 38% silver fluoride after tooth separation with orthodontic rubbers is a cheap, easy and quick method to directly diagnose caries and arrest multiple proximal active non-cavitated enamel lesions at a time in permanent teeth, while dark staining of these lesions is not or is barely visible in clinical follow-up examinations. For proximal dentin lesions without obvious cavitation, a re-application of SF may be useful, or other micro-invasive or traditional approaches may be necessary.

5. Patients' Perspective

Case 1

This patient was very surprised and disappointed that we found so many proximal lesions after the COVID-19 pandemic, as she did not have symptoms and was not expecting this at all in the control visit in February 2022. After experiencing local anesthesia and receiving fillings following this diagnostic visit, she and her mother were very satisfied that we could reduce the number of invasive treatments, and consequently the number of necessary dental visits, via application of SF.

Case 2

This patient did not care so much about the fact that he had caries and whether this meant that he might receive fillings or not, but rather cared about making multiple visits for their treatment. He and his mother were, therefore, highly satisfied with the technique, as we mainly could reduce the number of necessary dental visits. As they have quite a long drive to reach the clinic, irrespective of the duration of the dental visit, at least half a day is spent on attending treatment sessions. Despite the fact that some dentin lesions progressed (second quadrant), they were happy that invasive treatment was postponed.

Author Contributions: Conceptualization, J.S. methodology, J.S.; validation, J.S., E.E.A.A. and S.A.N.; formal analysis, J.S., E.E.A.A. and S.A.N.; investigation, E.E.A.A. and S.A.N.; resources J.S.; data curation, E.E.A.A. and S.A.N.; writing—original draft preparation, E.E.A.A. and S.A.N.; writing—review and editing, J.S.; visualization, E.E.A.A. and S.A.N.; supervision, J.S.; project administration, J.S.; All authors have read and agreed to the published version of the manuscript.

Funding: This research received no external funding.

Institutional Review Board Statement: Due to the nature of this article, no ethical approval was required.

Informed Consent Statement: Informed consent was obtained from parents/caregivers of all subjects involved.

Data Availability Statement: Data are fully presented in the article.

Acknowledgments: The authors want to thank the patients and caregivers for their openness to this innovative caries management approach and their time and consent for documentation (e.g., taking intraoral photos).

Conflicts of Interest: The authors declare no personal conflict of interest and no external funding for this project. It is worthwhile mentioning that the department of preventive and pediatric dentistry at the university medicine Greifswald has received partial funding from the company SDI for conducting other scientific projects.

References

1. Marsh, P. In Sickness and in Health—What Does the Oral Microbiome Mean to Us? An Ecological Perspective. *Adv. Dent. Res.* **2018**, *29*, 60–65. [CrossRef] [PubMed]
2. Kachuie, M.; Khoroushi, M. Prevention and treatment of white spot lesions in orthodontic patients. *Contemp. Clin. Dent.* **2017**, *8*, 11–19. [CrossRef] [PubMed]
3. Rechmann, P.; Kinsel, R.; Featherstone, J.D.B. Integrating Caries Management by Risk Assessment (CAMBRA) and Prevention Strategies Into the Contemporary Dental Practice. *Compend. Contin. Educ. Dent.* **2018**, *39*, 226.
4. Agarwal, D.; Machale, P.S.; Hegde-Shetiya, S. The Incipient Caries. *J. Contemp. Dent.* **2013**, *3*, 20–24. [CrossRef]
5. Mejàre, I.; Källestål, C.; Stenlund, H. Incidence and Progression of Approximal Caries from 11 to 22 Years of Age in Sweden: A Prospective Radiographic Study. *Caries Res.* **1999**, *33*, 93–100. [CrossRef]
6. Splieth, C.; Kanzow, P.; Wiegand, A.; Schmoeckel, J.; Jablonski-Momeni, A. How to intervene in the caries process: Proximal caries in adolescents and adults—A systematic review and meta-analysis. *Clin. Oral Investig.* **2020**, *24*, 1623–1636. [CrossRef]
7. Contreras, V.; Toro, M.J.; Elías-Boneta, A.R.; Encarnación-Burgos, A. Effectiveness of silver diamine fluoride in caries prevention and arrest: A systematic literature review. *Gen. Dent.* **2017**, *65*, 22–28.
8. Macey, R.; Walsh, T.; Riley, P.; Hogan, R.; Glenny, A.-M.; Worthington, H.V.; E Clarkson, J.; Ricketts, D. Transillumination and optical coherence tomography for the detection and diagnosis of enamel caries. *Cochrane Database Syst. Rev.* **2021**, *2021*, CD013855.
9. Shimada, Y.; Burrow, M.F.; Araki, K.; Zhou, Y.; Hosaka, K.; Sadr, A.; Yoshiyama, M.; Miyazaki, T.; Sumi, Y.; Tagami, J. 3D imaging of proximal caries in posterior teeth using optical coherence tomography. *Sci. Rep.* **2020**, *10*, 15754. [CrossRef]
10. Croll, T.P.; Berg, J. Delivery Methods of Silver Diammine Fluoride to Contacting Proximal Tooth Surfaces and History of Silver in Dentistry. *Compend. Contin. Educ. Dent.* **2020**, *41*, 84–89.
11. Oliveira, B.H.; Rajendra, A.; Veitz-Keenan, A.; Niederman, R. The Effect of Silver Diamine Fluoride in Preventing Caries in the Primary Dentition: A Systematic Review and Meta-Analysis. *Caries Res.* **2018**, *53*, 24–32. [CrossRef] [PubMed]
12. Gao, S.S.; Zhao, I.S.; Hiraishi, N.; Duangthip, D.; Mei, M.L.; Lo, E.C.; Chu, C.H. Clinical Trials of Silver Diamine Fluoride in Arresting Caries among Children: A Systematic Review. *JDR Clin. Trans. Res.* **2016**, *1*, 201–210. [CrossRef] [PubMed]
13. Punyanirun, K.; Yospiboonwong, T.; Kunapinun, T.; Thanyasrisung, P.; Trairatvorakul, C. Silver diamine fluoride remineralized artificial incipient caries in permanent teeth after bacterial pH-cycling in-vitro. *J. Dent.* **2018**, *69*, 55–59. [CrossRef] [PubMed]
14. Idoraşi, L.; Crăciunescu, E.L.; Stan, A.T.; Sinescu, C.; Chiş, A.C.; Onchiş-Moacă, D.; Romînu, M.; Negruţiu, M.L. Morphological aspects in remineralizing potential of Silver Diamine Fluoride. *Rom. J. Morphol. Embryol.* **2021**, *62*, 537–543. [CrossRef] [PubMed]
15. Riley, D.S.; Barber, M.S.; Kienle, G.S.; Aronson, J.K.; von Schoen-Angerer, T.; Tugwell, P.; Kiene, H.; Helfand, M.; Altman, D.G.; Sox, H.; et al. CARE guidelines for case reports: Explanation and elaboration document. *J. Clin. Epidemiol.* **2017**, *89*, 218–235. [CrossRef]
16. Young, D.A.; Nový, B.B.; Zeller, G.G.; Hale, R.; Hart, T.C.; Truelove, E.L.; Ekstrand, K.R.; Featherstone, J.D.; Fontana, M.; Ismail, A.; et al. The american dental association caries classification system for clinical practice: A report of the american dental association council on scientific affairs. *JADA* **2015**, *146*, 79–86.
17. Mialhe, F.; Pereira, A.; Meneghim, M.; Ambrosano, G.; Pardi, V. The relative diagnostic yields of clinical, FOTI and radiographic examinations for the detection of approximal caries in youngsters. *Indian. J. Dent. Res.* **2009**, *20*, 136–140. [CrossRef]
18. Ekstrand, K.R.; Zero, D.T.; Martignon, S.; Pitts, N.B. Detection, Assessment, Diagnosis and Monitoring of Caries. *Monogr. Oral Sci.* **2009**, *21*, 63–90. Available online: http://karger.com/books/book/chapter-pdf/2098567/000224213.pdf (accessed on 24 October 2023).
19. Crystal, Y.O.; Marghalani, A.A.; Ureles, S.D. Chairside Guide: Silver Diamine Fluoride in the Management of Dental Caries Lesions. *Pediatr. Dent.* **2017**, *39*, 135–145.
20. Young, D.A.; Quock, R.L.; Horst, J.; Kaur, R.; MacLean, J.K.; Frachella, J.C.; Duffin, S.; Semprum-Clavier, A.; Zandona, A.G. Clinical Instructions for Using Silver Diamine Fluoride (SDF) in Dental Caries Management. *Compend. Contin. Educ. Dent.* **2021**, *42*, 5–9.
21. Hassan, M.; Bakhurji, E.; Alsheikh, R. Application of Er,Cr:YSGG laser versus photopolymerization after silver diamine fluoride in primary teeth. *Sci. Rep.* **2021**, *11*, 20780. [CrossRef] [PubMed]
22. Ruff, R.R.; Whittemore, R.; Grochecki, M.; Bateson, J.; Barry Godín, T.J. Silver diamine fluoride and oral health-related quality of life: A review and network meta-analysis. *PLoS ONE* **2022**, *17*, e0261627. [CrossRef] [PubMed]
23. Mitchell, C.; Gross, A.J.; Milgrom, P.; Mancl, L.; Prince, D.B. Silver diamine fluoride treatment of active root caries lesions in older adults: A case series. *J. Dent.* **2021**, *105*, 103561. [CrossRef]
24. Keys, T.; Burrow, M.F.; Rajan, S.; Rompre, P.; Doméjean, S.; Muller-Bolla, M.; Manton, D.J. Carious lesion management in children and adolescents by Australian dentists. *Aust. Dent. J.* **2019**, *64*, 282–292. [CrossRef]
25. Daruich, P.; Brizuela, M. *Remineralization of Initial Carious Lesions*; StatPearls: Treasure Island, FL, USA, 2022.

26. Schwendicke, F.; Meyer-Lueckel, H.; Stolpe, M.; Dörfer, C.E.; Paris, S. Costs and Effectiveness of Treatment Alternatives forProximal Caries Lesions. *PLoS ONE* **2014**, *1*, E86992.
27. Melo, M.; Pascual, A.; Camps, I.; Ata-Ali, F.; Ata-Ali, J. Combined Near-Infrared Light Transillumination and Direct Digital Radiography Increases Diagnostic in Approximal Caries. *Sci. Rep.* **2019**, *9*, 14224. [CrossRef]
28. Yalçın Yeler, D.; Koraltan, M. Diagnostic accuracy of five different techniques for detection of approximal caries. *Acta Odontol. Turc.* **2017**, *35*, 9–16. [CrossRef]
29. Alammar, R.; Sadaf, D. Accurate detection of non-cavitated proximal caries in posterior permanent teeth: An in vivo study. *Risk Manag. Healthc. Policy* **2020**, *13*, 1431–1436. [CrossRef]
30. Schwendicke, F.; Göstemeyer, G. Conventional bitewing radiography. *Clin. Dent. Rev.* **2020**, *4*, 22–30. [CrossRef]
31. Chray, M.; Khorn, S.; Da, S.; Turton, B.; Durward, C. Pilot evaluation of the therapeutic effect of Silver Diamine Fluoride (SDF) in Arresting dental caries in the primary teeth of Cambodian slum children. In Proceedings of the 11th International Dentistry Scientific Meeting (IDSM 2017), Central Jakarta, Indonesia, 16–17 September 2017; Atlantis Press: Amsterdam, The Netherlands, 2018; pp. 125–133.
32. Amaechi, B.T. Remineralization Therapies for Initial Caries Lesions. *Curr. Oral Health Rep.* **2015**, *2*, 95–101. [CrossRef]
33. Dorri, M.; Dunne, S.M.; Walsh, T.; Schwendicke, F. Micro-invasive interventions for managing proximal dental decay in primary and permanent teeth. *Cochrane Database Syst. Rev.* **2015**, *11*, CD010431. [CrossRef] [PubMed]
34. Sorkhdini, P.; Crystal, Y.O.; Tang, Q.; Lippert, F. The effect of silver diamine fluoride on the remineralization of early enamel carious lesions under pH-cycling conditions. *JADA Found. Sci.* **2022**, *1*, 100006. [CrossRef]
35. Kidd, E.A.M.; Fejerskov, O. What Constitutes Dental Caries? Histopathology of Carious Enamel and Dentin Related to the Action of Cariogenic Biofilms. *J. Dent. Res.* **2004**, *83*, 35–38. [CrossRef] [PubMed]
36. Merchant, A.T. Flossing for 2 Weeks Reduces Microbes Associated with Oral Disease. *J. Evid. Based Dent. Pract.* **2009**, *9*, 223–224. [CrossRef] [PubMed]
37. Corby, P.M.; Biesbrock, A.; Bartizek, R.; Corby, A.L.; Monteverde, R.; Ceschin, R.; Bretz, W.A. Treatment Outcomes of Dental Flossing in Twins: Molecular Analysis of the Interproximal Microflora | Enhanced Reader. *J. Periodontol.* **2008**, *79*, 1426–1433. [CrossRef]
38. Ashkenazi, M.; Bidoosi, M.; Levin, L. Factors associated with reduced compliance of children to dental preventive measures. *Odontology* **2012**, *100*, 241–248. [CrossRef]
39. Ekstrand, K.R.; Bakhshandeh, A.; Martignon, S.; Ekstrand, K. Treatment of Proximal Superficial Caries Lesions on Primary Molar Teeth with Resin Infiltration and Fluoride Varnish versus Fluoride Varnish Only: Efficacy after 1 Year. *Caries Res.* **2010**, *44*, 41–46. [CrossRef]
40. Altarabulsi, M.B.; Alkilzy, M.; Petrou, M.A.; Splieth, C. Aus der Abteilung für präventive Zahnmedizin und Kinderzahnheilkunde Clinical Applicability, Safety and Effect of Resin Infiltration for Proximal Caries. *Eur. J. Paediatr. Dent.* **2012**, *15*, 39–44.
41. Alkilzy, M.; Berndt, C.; Splieth, C.H. Sealing proximal surfaces with polyurethane tape: Three-year evaluation. *Clin. Oral Investig.* **2011**, *15*, 879–884. [CrossRef]
42. Chen, Y.; Chen, D.; Lin, H. Infiltration and sealing for managing non-cavitated proximal lesions: A systematic review and meta-analysis. *BMC Oral Health* **2020**, *21*, 13. [CrossRef]
43. Diab, E.; Hesse, D.; Bonifacio, C.C. A retrospective clinical study on the resin infiltration of proximal caries lesions: The operator's effect. *Eur. Arch. Paediatr. Dent.* **2021**, *22*, 879–885. [CrossRef] [PubMed]
44. Crystal, Y.O.; Niederman, R. Evidence-Based Dentistry Update on Silver Diamine Fluoride. *Dent. Clin. N. Am.* **2019**, *63*, 45–68. [CrossRef] [PubMed]
45. Crystal, Y.O.; Janal, M.N.; Hamilton, D.S.; Niederman, R. Parental perceptions and acceptance of silver diamine fluoride staining. *JADA* **2017**, *148*, 510–518. [CrossRef] [PubMed]

Disclaimer/Publisher's Note: The statements, opinions and data contained in all publications are solely those of the individual author(s) and contributor(s) and not of MDPI and/or the editor(s). MDPI and/or the editor(s) disclaim responsibility for any injury to people or property resulting from any ideas, methods, instructions or products referred to in the content.

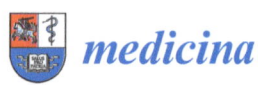

Systematic Review

Cost-Effectiveness of Treatment Decisions for Early Childhood Caries in Infants and Toddlers: A Systematic Review

Thomas Gerhard Wolf [1,2,*] and Guglielmo Campus [3]

[1] Department of Restorative, Preventive and Pediatric Dentistry, University of Bern, Freiburgstrasse 7, 3010 Bern, Switzerland

[2] Department of Periodontology and Operative Dentistry, University Medical Center of the Johannes Gutenberg University Mainz, 55116 Mainz, Germany

[3] Department of Surgery, Microsurgery and Medicine Sciences, School of Dentistry, University of Sassari, Viale San Pietro, 07100 Sassari, Italy; guglielmo.campus@unibe.ch

* Correspondence: thomas.wolf@unibe.ch; Tel.: +41-31-684-06-50

Abstract: *Background and Objectives:* Early childhood caries (ECC) is a multifactorial, biofilm-mediated, sugar-related, dynamic disease of primary dental hard tissues occurring in varying degrees of severity in infants and toddlers. Untreated ECC may lead to pain, infections, and severe systemic complications. The aim of this study was to systematically review and evaluate the scientific evidence on the cost-effectiveness of treatment decisions in ECC in infants and toddlers. *Materials and Methods:* Observational epidemiological studies, i.e., cohort studies, case–control studies, and randomized controlled trials, reporting cost-effectiveness of treatment decisions in ECC in infants and toddlers were included in the systematic review following the PRISMA guidelines. Using an ad hoc search with search terms or keywords (MeSH), electronic databases Embase, MEDLINE via PubMed, Scopus, and gray literature were searched. *Results:* The search identified 494 articles, of which 446 remained after removing duplicates. A total of 417 articles were excluded after title and abstract evaluation; 29 full-text articles were screened for eligibility, and five articles were discarded. Twenty-four full-text articles were included in the systematic review, assigning 17 to prevention and seven to restoration. Results were heterogeneous; comparability of included studies is difficult because of the different methodologies used. Conflicting efficacies were demonstrated for different interventions implemented, and cost-effectiveness data were documented. *Conclusions:* Socioeconomic, cultural, and ethnic differences must be considered when comparing conditions in terms of cost-effectiveness. A paradigm shift from surgical towards preventive treatment decisions can be observed. Cost-effectiveness studies on therapies for ECC in infants and toddlers are needed to identify the best practice approach and the most cost-effective therapy decisions.

Keywords: cost-effectiveness; early childhood caries; infant; treatment; toddler; young children

Citation: Wolf, T.G.; Campus, G. Cost-Effectiveness of Treatment Decisions for Early Childhood Caries in Infants and Toddlers: A Systematic Review. *Medicina* **2023**, *59*, 1865. https://doi.org/10.3390/medicina59101865

Academic Editor: Edgaras Stankevičius

Received: 12 September 2023
Revised: 9 October 2023
Accepted: 14 October 2023
Published: 20 October 2023

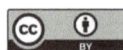

Copyright: © 2023 by the authors. Licensee MDPI, Basel, Switzerland. This article is an open access article distributed under the terms and conditions of the Creative Commons Attribution (CC BY) license (https://creativecommons.org/licenses/by/4.0/).

1. Introduction

Early childhood caries (ECC) has gained importance in the past decade worldwide [1–6]. ECC, in the past also occasionally called as "baby bottle syndrome", "breastfeeding caries", "bottle mouth caries", "rampant caries", or "wild caries", is characterized by carious lesions that produce an invasion of the dental hard tissue on deciduous tooth surfaces and occur within the first three years of life in infants and toddlers [1–6]. Dental caries remains the most common disease of mankind and plays an important role in ensuring good oral and general health [6]. Early childhood caries can be differentiated into three levels of severity, with the mild/moderate form often occurring between the ages of 2 and 5 years, where it is also stated to occur up to 71 months, which corresponds to under 6 years [1–7]. The mild/moderate form often occurs between the ages of 2 and 5 years on deciduous molars and/or incisors (ECC type I), the moderate to severe form occurs on maxillary (maxillary) incisors with caries-free mandibular (mandibular) incisors often shortly after deciduous tooth eruption (ECC type II), and the severe form involves almost all deciduous teeth including the mandibular incisors in predominantly 3- to 5-year-old infants (EDD type III) [1]. Prevalence is reported between 5% and 20% in Germany [8–10] and between 3% and 45% worldwide [11] in epidemiological studies. In the past, early childhood caries could only be diagnosed with the dental screening examination for children beginning at 30 months of age; however, between 7% and 20% of children already have early childhood caries at this time [12]. An association of population strata with both low social status and low education levels can be observed, with 2% of children already showing 52% of caries [13]. However, middle class populations were also clustered in early childhood caries due to misinformation about causes of the disease [14].

The causes for the occurrence of early childhood caries are manifold. These include both behavioral and social risk factors [15]. In addition to a possible transmission of cariogenic microbes from mother to child, e.g., by licking the bottle or the pacifier, the consumption of sugary and acidic foods or frequent snacks such as the consumption of sweets are also significant factors. In addition to nocturne bottle sucking, inadequate oral and dental hygiene as well as irregular intake of fluoridation measures for prophylaxis are also significant for the development and progression of the disease [15].

The possible consequences of early childhood caries are pain and multiple inflammations with an early loss of milk teeth and thus resulting in both aesthetic and functional impairment [2–6]. However, it can also lead to possible damage to the germs of permanent teeth, which is often accompanied by impaired tooth eruption, developmental disorders of the upper and lower jaw, impaired speech development, insufficient nutritional behavior, and dysfunctional chewing or swallowing ability [2–6]. In addition to the psychosocial developmental deficits caused by the caries that have occurred or the loss of teeth, especially in the visible anterior region, a lack of compliance for future visits to the dentist often develops [15]. While mild to moderate early childhood caries (ECC type I–II) is often still feasible with premedication (midazolam), nitrous oxide, or behavioral guidance/hypnosis, in the case of severe early childhood caries (ECC type III), often only remediation under ITN (intubation anesthesia, general anesthesia) remains due to the intensive and time-consuming treatment with simultaneous frequent lack of compliance [2–6]. However, the dangers of both sedation and general anesthesia due to dental caries disease must not be underestimated under any circumstances, because such sedative/anesthetic treatments pose an enormous health risk for an infant or young child and not infrequently lead to complications and even death [16,17].

Intervention strategies with in-depth diagnostics and preventive as well as therapeutic measures are necessary [18–20]. Above all, prevention in combination with an interdisciplinary approach should enable dentists to work better with family doctors, pediatricians, gynecologists, as well as midwives in this area to prevent caries as early as possible. In order to detect and diagnose the disease even before group or individual prophylaxis is reached at preschool age, the benefits catalog of the statutory health insurance in Germany was expanded about four years ago to include three additional dental screening examinations for toddlers from 6 months to 33 months of age [15]. The early detection examinations are to take place between the 6th and 9th (FU1), the 10th and 20th (FU2), and from the 21st month of life (FU3). The dental screening examinations focus on the causal development of caries and therefore include, in addition to a detailed examination of the child, counseling of the parents with specific instructions for regular, daily tooth brushing and enamel hardening with fluoride varnish twice per calendar half-year, to which toddlers are legally entitled.

Cost efficiency has become an enormously important aspect of public health care. Cost-effectiveness analysis is defined as "a way to examine both the costs and health outcomes of one or more interventions. It compares an intervention to another intervention (or the status quo) by estimating how much it costs to gain a unit of a health outcome, like a life year gained or a death prevented" [21]. By means of cost-effectiveness analyses of different therapies, additional information can be obtained in the sense of the cost-effectiveness requirement of the statutory or state health insurance system, in which every medical treatment must be sufficient, appropriate, and economical, which can influence participative decision-making between dentist and patient (or child accompanied by parents). To date, few systematic reviews have focused on cost-effectiveness in children. To the best of our knowledge, no systematic review for cost-effectiveness of treatment decisions for ECC in infants and young children has been conducted.

Therefore, the aim of this study is to systematically review and summarize research findings on the cost-effectiveness of treatment decisions for early childhood caries in infants and toddlers.

2. Materials and Methods

2.1. Protocol and Registration

This systematic review was registered with the International Center for Open Science (Center for Open Science, 210 Ridge McIntire Road, Suite 500, Charlottesville, VA, USA) and addresses the cost-effectiveness of treatment decisions of early childhood caries in infants and toddlers and includes in vivo studies from birth to 71 months [22]. Data collected are in accordance with the most recent Preferred Reporting Items for Systematic Reviews and Meta-Analyses Statement (PRISMA 2020) guidelines for reporting systematic reviews of health care interventions [23].

2.2. Inclusion and Exclusion Criteria

The inclusion criteria were as follows: observational epidemiologic studies (cohort studies, case–control studies, and randomized controlled trials) that reported on the cost-effectiveness of treatment decisions in early childhood caries in infants and toddlers. Studies that evaluated cost-effectiveness using cost-effectiveness modeling (e.g., Markov model) or that only performed cost simulation without the direct link to clinical intervention were explicitly excluded.

The following PICO questions (population, intervention, comparison, and outcome) were formulated [24]:

- P = infants and toddlers aged 0 to 71 months;
- I = treatments for early childhood caries (ECC);
- C = cost-effectiveness of treatment decisions;
- O = summary or relative order/priority of the strategies.

Due to the great heterogeneity in the study and the types of dental materials used in this research area, no common comparator was defined for the included studies. Nevertheless, all studies were included and comparatively evaluated regarding the outcome "cost-effectiveness of treatment decisions".

The SPIDER (sample, phenomenon of interest, design, evaluation, research) method was also used to create the search strategy [25,26]. Thus, the following conceptualizations were included in conjunction with the concept of "Therapeutic Decision Making":

- S = population*, subject*, high risk*, group*, age group*.
- PI = The terms "decision making, cost, cost-effec*, beneficial, prevention, treatment, caries, dental caries" are used to evaluate the concept of "treatment decision making".
- D = Quantitative original publications are considered.
- E = The search strategy is not restricted regarding the evaluation (E) of the publication since there are probably few comprehensive data on this area.
- R = RCT, cohort studies, and case–control studies are the studies of first choice. No time restriction is applied as an exclusion criterion. Publications in English, German, French, or Italian will be considered.

2.3. Data Sources, Search Strategy and Study Selection

Detailed search terms and a search strategy were created using Boolean operators. An ad hoc literature search was performed using search terms, keywords (MeSH—medical subject headings), in the electronic databases MEDLINE via PubMed, Embase, Scopus, and Open Grey Literature (https://www.opengrey.eu, accessed on 14 July 2023). The last search for all electronic databases took place on 14 July 2023. In addition, a hand search was performed. Articles in English, German, French, or Italian were considered. Furthermore, the references of all the included studies were also hand-searched. The electronic databases were searched according to their advanced search syntax using a search strategy identical for the three databases. Duplicates were removed from the literature search results. Cross-references were also made using the bibliographies of the full-text articles. Data were reported according to the updated Preferred Reporting Items for Systematic Reviews and Meta-Analyses 2020 (PRISMA) guidelines [23]. The PRISMA checklist is available in the Supplementary Material (Figure S1). The search strategy included search terms for each selected electronic database. For MEDLINE via Pubmed, the following search terms were used: ((("carie" [All Fields] OR "dental caries" [MeSH Terms] OR ("dental" [All Fields] AND "caries" [All Fields]) OR "dental caries" [All Fields] OR "caries" [All Fields]) AND (("manage" [All Fields] OR "managed" [All Fields] OR "management s" [All Fields] OR "managements" [All Fields] OR "manager" [All Fields] OR "manager s" [All Fields] OR "managers" [All Fields] OR "manages" [All Fields] OR "managing" [All Fields] OR "managment" [All Fields] OR "organization and administration" [MeSH Terms] OR ("organization" [All Fields] AND "administration" [All Fields]) OR "organization and administration" [All Fields] OR "management" [All Fields] OR "disease management" [MeSH Terms] OR ("disease" [All Fields] AND "management" [All Fields]) OR "disease management" [All Fields]) AND ("infant" [MeSH Terms] OR "infant" [MeSH Terms:noexp] OR "child, preschool" [MeSH Terms] OR "child" [MeSH Terms:noexp])) AND ("infant" [MeSH Terms] OR "infant" [MeSH Terms:noexp] OR "child, preschool" [MeSH Terms] OR "child" [MeSH Terms:noexp]) AND (((("carie" [All Fields] OR "dental caries" [MeSH Terms] OR ("dental" [All Fields] AND "caries" [All Fields]) OR "dental caries" [All Fields] OR "caries" [All Fields]) AND ("clinical trial" [Publication Type] OR "randomized controlled trial" [Publication Type]) AND ("infant" [MeSH Terms] OR "child" [MeSH Terms:noexp] OR "infant" [MeSH Terms:noexp] OR "child, preschool" [MeSH Terms])) OR ("early" [All Fields] AND ("childhood" [All Fields] OR "childhoods" [All Fields]) AND ("carie" [All Fields] OR "dental caries" [MeSH Terms] OR ("dental" [All Fields] AND "caries" [All Fields]) OR "dental caries" [All Fields] OR "caries" [All Fields]))) AND ("infant" [MeSH Terms] OR "infant" [MeSH Terms:noexp] OR "child, preschool" [MeSH Terms] OR "child" [MeSH Terms:noexp])) AND ("infant" [MeSH Terms] OR "infant" [MeSH Terms:noexp] OR "child, preschool" [MeSH Terms] OR "child" [MeSH Terms:noexp]) AND (("cost benefit analysis" [MeSH Terms] OR ("cost benefit" [All Fields] AND "analysis" [All Fields]) OR "cost benefit analysis" [All Fields] OR ("economic" [All Fields] AND "evaluation" [All Fields]) OR "economic evaluation" [All Fields]) AND ("infant" [MeSH Terms] OR "infant" [MeSH Terms:noexp] OR "child, preschool" [MeSH Terms] OR "child" [MeSH Terms:noexp]))) AND (allinfant [Filter] OR infant [Filter] OR preschoolchild [Filter] OR child [Filter]).

The titles and abstracts of all the identified studies were first reviewed independently by the authors. Abstracts were assessed if the title indicated possible inclusion. After careful review of the abstracts, those manuscripts that were eligible for review and available in full text were selected. Full texts were then assessed and reviewed independently for content and inclusion in the study. In case of disagreement, there was an opportunity for agreement on inclusion of studies or data extraction by consulting with an additional researcher. Microsoft Excel spreadsheets (Microsoft Corporation, Redmont, WA, USA) were used for recording and data extraction. They were completed so that each eligible study was assigned a study ID that included the author's name, year of publication, and country of study conduct.

The following data were also extracted:
- Setting: duration of study, site of data collection or examination or treatment, number of patients, age of patients, type of treatment, type of control group, number of teeth or lesions, if any, follow-up, cost of treatment, cost of control group, clinical outcome;

- Materials: prevention or restoration (classification, name);
- Methodological aspects: study design, evaluation criteria, for e.g., restoration survival or intervention.

2.4. Data Collection and Evaluation of Study Quality

Data collection and synthesis were performed using an ad hoc designed extraction table without masking the name of the journal, title, or even authors. Studies were classified chronologically according to their country of study conduct, number of study participants, location (e.g., practice/clinic) of study conduct, age of study participants, and study quality assessment. Furthermore, included studies were classified into two main groups of prevention according to their primary outcome [18,27–41] and restoration [42–48] with different subgroups divided at prevention (outreach/education/education, sealing, fluoride varnish, and silver diamine fluoride (SDF) and atraumatic restorative treatment (ART) as well as restoration (filling and crown). For ease of synthesis and clarity, the results were summarized in tables. Accordingly, for each article, these data were queried and recorded when available: (a) authors, year of publication, source of publication, site of study conduct, duration of study in months, site of study conduct (practice/clinic), number of participants, age of participants in years, and quality assessment (risk of bias) of studies, (b) study design and treatment (intervention) and control groups, and (c) cost of treatment (intervention), cost of control group, and clinical outcome. Areas (b) and (c) were respectively divided into prevention (information/education/education, sealing, fluoride varnish, and silver diamine fluoride (SDF) and atraumatic restorative treatment (ART)) and restoration (filling and crown).

An individual quality assessment tool developed by the National Heart, Lung, and Blood Institute of the National Institute of Health (Bethesda, Maryland, USA) for observational cohorts, case–control study, and controlled intervention studies was used (Study Quality Assessment Tools, NHLBI, NHI; https://www.nhlbi.nih.gov/health-topics/study-quality-assessment-tools, last accessed 12 September 2023). The quality of the studies was assessed according to the following criteria: low/poor quality ("poor"): 0–6, adequate quality ("fair"): 7–11, and good quality ("good"). The quality assessment of the studies is intended to provide information on the internal validity of a study and to consider the risk of bias through critical evaluation.

3. Results

The search identified a total of 494 articles; 446 were selected after duplicates were removed and 417 articles were excluded after review or evaluation of title and abstract. The list of excluded studies after initial review can be found in Supplementary Materials (Table S1). Twenty-nine articles were reviewed for eligibility by full text, of which five articles were discarded after review of the full text. No articles were added by hand search, i.e., without Boolean search terms via electronic databases. There were 24 full-text articles included in the review work, of which 17 articles were assigned to prevention and 7 to restoration. The flowchart of the search can be seen in Supplementary Materials (Figure S2).

There were ultimately 24 articles included in this systematic review, with two articles each reporting the same study [34,49] as well as [34,48]. While the articles [34,49] were about similar results, the articles [43,48] represented the baseline study [43] and the follow-up study with final clinical trial results [48]. Of the 24 articles included in the systematic review, 17 articles could be classified as prevention [18,27–41,49]. Seven studies were classified as restoration [42–48]. All included studies were published in the last decade [18,27–49]. Most of the included articles (12 studies) and thus half of the articles were published in the last 3 years from 2020 to 2023 [18,33–41,48,49].

Study Characteristics

The included studies were a total of seven retrospective cohort studies [27,31,33,37,39, 41,42], one uncontrolled [29], one cohort study [23], and randomized controlled trials [18,28,

30,32,34–36,38,40,43–49] (Table 1). The summaries of the selected studies are presented in Table 2. Most studies were conducted in the United Kingdom of Great Britain and Northern Ireland [28,29,31,34,35,47,49], the United States [27,28,37,42], and Brazil [32,43,46,48]. Sixteen studies were conducted in public health facilities or schools [18,27–32,35,36,38,40,41,43,44,48,49], one study in a specialized dental practice [42], one study in a day care center [46], four studies in general or private dental practices [33,34,45,47], one study in an outpatient clinic or operating room [37], and one study that examined dental services only [46]. Of the included studies, a total of 14 were considered "good" [27,28,31,32,35,36,40,41,43–48] and ten studies rated as "fair" [18,29,30,33,34,37–39,42,49] (Tables 2 and 3).

In the prevention domain, there were one study each on outreach/education and sealant, eight studies on fluoride varnish [18,28,29,33,35,38,41,49], and seven studies on silver diamine fluoride (SDF) and atraumatic restorative treatment (ART) [30–33,36,39,40]. In the restorative field, three studies were on filling [43,46,48] and four on crown [42,44,45,47]. Due to the heterogeneity in both the methodology used on treatment and control groups and the different clinical outcomes, a further synthesis of the results on cost-effectiveness (Table 4) of individual techniques or methods is not possible. In total, the 24 articles included 77,546 children in the systematic review. Eighteen studies had a sample size of more than 100 participants [18,27–31,33–35,37–39,41,43,44,46–48]. Most studies have been conducted in children between the ages of 3 and 7 years.

Table 1. Synthesis of the studies included in the systematic review with information on ID no., authors, year of publication, country of study conduct, study design, treatment (intervention), and control group divided into prevention (information/education/education, sealing, fluoride varnish, and silver diamine fluoride (SDF) and atraumatic restorative treatment (ART)) and restoration (filling and crown).

ID	Authors	Year	Country	Study Design	Treatment	Control
					Prevention	
					Education	
1	Nowak et al. [27]	2014	USA	Retrospective cohort study	Early starters (age at first visit to dentist < 4 years)	Late starters (age at first dental visit > 4 years)
					Sealing	
2	Halasa-Rappel et al. [37]	2021	USA	5-year retrospective cohort study	Pitting and fissure sealing (sealed)	No pitting and fissure sealing (not sealed)
					Fluoride varnish	
3	Zaror et al. [18]	2020	Chile	Two-year follow-up, triple-blind, randomized, controlled trial	Fluoride varnish	Control (placebo)
4	McMahon et al. [35]	2020	UK	Double-blind, two-arm, randomized, controlled trial	Fluoride varnish application plus treatment-as-usual (TAU) and Childsmile program interventions	TAU and Childsmile program interventions
5	Buckingham & John [29]	2017	UK	Uncontrolled cohort study	Fluoride varnish applications (one, two, and three)	
6	Tickle et al. [28]	2017	UK	Two-arm, randomized, controlled, parallel-group study	Intervention: composite, fluoride varnish 22,600 (ppm); toothpaste at 1450 ppm; and 50-mL standardized, evidence-based prevention counseling at semiannual intervals for 3 years	The control group received prevention counseling alone
7	Homer et al. [33]	2020	UK	Three-arm, randomized, controlled, parallel-group study	Conventional with best practice prevention (C + P), C + P (e.g., local anesthesia, removal of carious tissue and restoration)	Biological with best practice prevention (B + P): B + P (e.g., partial/no removal and restoration of carious tissue) or best practice prevention alone (PA)

Table 1. Cont.

ID	Authors	Year	Country	Study Design	Treatment	Control
8	Maguire et al. [49]	202	UK	Multicenter, three-arm, participant-randomized, controlled, parallel-group study	(1) Best practice prevention (local anesthesia, removal of carious tissue, placement of fillings)	(2) Best practice prevention (sealing of caries, selective removal of carious tissue, and fissure sealing) and (3) best practice prevention alone (dietary and toothbrushing recommendations, topical fluoride, and fissure sealing of permanent teeth)
9	Effenberger et al. [45]	2022	South Africa	Multicenter, two-arm, single-blind, cluster-randomized, controlled superiority trial with parallel groups	Fluoride varnish every 3 months and supervised brushing with fluoridated toothpaste	No fluoride varnish, supervised brushing with fluoride toothpaste
10	Nantanee & Sriratanaban [41]	202	Thailand	Retro and prospective cohort study	Fluoride varnish	
				Silver diamine fluoride (SDF) and atraumatic restorative treatment (ART)		
11	Nguyen et al. [39]	2022	Australia	Australian single cohort study	SDF + standard support	SDF—without standard support
12	Tonmukayakul & Arrow [30]	201	Australia	Pragmatic, randomized, controlled trial	Atraumatic restorative treatment (ART)	Standard care (SC)
13	Bottega et al. [32]	2018	Brazil	Randomized, descriptive, and analytic clinical trial	Papacarie group (caries removal with the chemical-mechanical method—Papacarie gel)	Drill group (caries removal with the traditional method—drilling)
14	Aly et al. [47]	202	Egypt	Randomized, two-arm, parallel-group, controlled trial (allocation ratio 1:1)	Silver-modified atraumatic restorative treatment (SMART)	Atraumatic restorative treatment (ART)
15	Davis et al. [33]	2020	USA	Retrospective cohort study	Silver diamine fluoride (SDF)	No SDF
16	BaniHani et al. [31]	201	UK	Retrospective (cost-effectiveness)/prospective cohort study (patient + caregiver acceptance/outcome)	Non-selective removal of hard dentin with/without pulp therapy	Selective removal of solid dentin and the Hall technique
17	Elhennawy et al. [36]	2021	Germany	Two-arm, single-blind, randomized, controlled superiority trial with parallel groups	Selective caries removal (SE)	Stepwise caries removal (SW)

Table 1. Cont.

ID	Authors	Year	Country	Study Design	Treatment	Control
					Restoration	
					Filling	
18	de Moura et al. [46]	2019	Brazil	Randomized controlled trial	Vitro Molar®	Ketac Molar®
19	Olegário et al. [43]	201	Brazil	Three-arm, parallel, randomized clinical trial	G1-GC Fumi IX Gold Label 9 (GC Corp)	G2-Vitro Molar (DFL) and G3-Maxxion R (FGM)
20	Olegário et al. [48]	2020	Brazil	Double-blind (participants and evaluators), randomized, three-arm (1:1:1 allocation) clinical trial	G1-GC Fumi IX Gold Label 9 (GC Corp)	G2-Vitro Molar (DFL) and G3-Maxxion R (FGM)
					Crown	
21	Schwendicke et al. [43]	2018	Germany	Randomized study	Hall technology (HT)	Non-restorative cavity control (NRCC) and conventional carious tissue removal and restoration (CR)
22	Elamin et al. [45]	201	Sudan	Randomized clinical trial	Preformed metal crowns (PMCs) placed with conventional techniques (CTs)	PMCs placed by the biological reverberation technique (HT)
23	Schwendicke et al. [47]	2019	UK	Randomized, controlled, split-mouth practice trial	Hall technology (HT)	Conventional removal and restoration of carious tissue (CR)
24	Holsinger et al. [42]	201	USA	Retrospective cohort study	Zircon crowns	

Table 2. Studies included in the systematic review with information on ID number, authors, year of publication, source of publication, site of study conduct, duration of study in months, site of study conduct (practice/clinic), number of participants, age of participants in years, and quality assessment (risk of bias) of the studies. The NIH quality assessment tool rates the observational, cross-sectional, and controlled intervention studies as good, fair (adequate), or poor.

N	Authors	Year	Source	Country	Duration (Months)	Practice/Clinic	n (Participants)	Age (Years)	Quality
1	Nowak et al. [27]	2014	Pediatric Dentistry	USA	96	20 dental care centers	N = 42,532 (n = 17,040 early starters, first dental visit < 4 years old, n = 25,492 late starters, first dental visit > 4 years old).	0 to 7	Good

Table 2. *Cont.*

N	Authors	Year	Source	Country	Duration (Months)	Practice/Clinic	n (Participants)	Age (Years)	Quality
2	Holsinger et al. [42]	201	Pediatric Dentistry	USA	6-37, 6-8 (n = 14), 14 (n = 30)	Pediatric dental practice	18 from 53 children (57 crowns)	2 to 6	Fair
3	Tickle et al. [28]	2016	Health Technology Assessment	Northern Ireland, UK	36	22 NHS dental practices in Northern Ireland and the United Kingdom	1096 from 1248 children	2 to 3	Good
4	Buckingham & John [29]	201	British Dental Journal	UK	1	Two sites in Southampton and Oxfordshire and three in Portsmouth	458 (589)	4 to 7	Fair
5	Olegário et al. [43]	2017	Journal of Dentistry	Brazil	2, 6, and 12 months	Public schools in the city	150 milk molars in 150 children	4 to 8	Good
6	Tonmukayakul & Arrow [30]	201	Community Dental and Oral Epidemiology	Australia	12	Real-world practice of public health service	254 children	<5	Fair
7	BaniHani et al. [31]	2018	Caries Research	UK	77	Two dental clinics	Retrospectively n = 246 (114 conventional, 132 organic), prospectively n = 110	4 to 9	Good
8	Bottega et al. [32]	201	Scientific Reports	Brazil	1	Municipal schools	24 (12 girls/12 boys), 48 restorations	5.9	Good
9	Schwendicke et al. [44]	2018	Journal of Dentistry	Germany	30	Department of Preventive and Pediatric Dentistry, University Medical Center Greifswald, Germany	142 from 169 children	3 to 8	Good
10	de Moura et al. [46]	201	Brazilian Oral Research	Brazil	1	Day care centers	243 (728 restorations) included, 1077 preschoolers participated with 21,540 teeth evaluated	2 to 6	Good
11	Elamin et al. [45]	2019	Plos One	Sudan	24	General dental practices	86 children with 109 PMCs (HT) and 78 children with 103 PMCs (CT)	5 to 8	Good

Table 2. *Cont.*

N	Authors	Year	Source	Country	Duration (Months)	Practice/Clinic	n (Participants)	Age (Years)	Quality
12	Schwendicke et al. [47]	2019	Journal of Dental Research	Scotland, UK	60	17 general dental practices in Scotland in rural, urban, and mixed locations	264 milk molars (132 children)	4 to 9 (10)	Good
13	Davis et al. [33]	2020	The Journal of Clinical Pediatric Dentistry	USA	12	Documentation/patient records of one practice, two private practices	104 (SDF), 250 (non-SDF)	6	Fair
14	Homer et al. [34]	2020	BMC Oral Health	UK	35.5 (min 23, max 36)	General dental practices in England, Scotland, and Wales	1058 from 1144 children	3 to 7	Fair
15	Maguire et al. [49]	2020	Health Technology Assessment	UK	33.8 (23.8–36.7)	72 primary care dental practices	1058 from 1144 children	3 to 7	Fair
16	Nowak et al. [27]	2020	Community Oral Health	UK	24 (6 month interval)	Dental practice, dental outpatient clinics in hospitals	1150 of 1284 children (n = 577 FV, n = 573 TAU, 10% drop-out).	3.5	Good
17	Olegário et al. [48]	2020	Journal of Dentistry	Brazil	24	27 public schools in the city	150 out of 1200 children evaluated	4 to 8	Good
18	Zaror et al. [18]	2020	Journal of Dentistry	Chile	24	Public rural preschools in areas without access to fluoridated water	275	2 to 3	Fair
19	Elhennawy et al. [36]	2021	Clinical Oral Investigations	Germany	24	Dental Clinic of the Charité—Universitätsmedizin Berlin, Germany	74 children (1 molar/child)	3 to 9	Good
20	Halasa-Rappel et al. [37]	2021	Journal of the American Dental Association	USA	60	Outpatient clinic or operating room	390 children (1884 milk molars)	<6	Fair
21	Effenberger et al. [38]	2022	Community Dental and Oral Epidemiology	South Africa	24	Two schools in the township	513 (from 717)	4 to 8	Fair
22	Nguyen et al. [39]	2022	Australian Dental Journal	Australia	6	Examination of dental services	102 Victorian children	2 to 10	Fair

Table 2. *Cont.*

N	Authors	Year	Source	Country	Duration (Months)	Practice/Clinic	n (Participants)	Age (Years)	Quality
23	Aly et al. [40]	2023	Journal of Dentistry	Egypt	12	Outpatient Clinic of the Department of Pediatric Dentistry and Public Dental Health	67 (SMART group (n = 34, 59 molars) and ART control group (n = 33, 60 molars)).	5 to 9	Good
24	Nantanee & Sriratanaban [41]	202	Community Dental and Oral Epidemiology	Thailand	9–12, 18, 24 and 30	Two randomly selected districts in each of Thailand's three provinces	460 children	9 to 30 months (19.2 ± 1.7 month	Good

Table 3. Study quality assessment tool NHLBI, NHI; https://www.nhlbi.nih.gov/health-topics/study-quality-assessment-tools; last accessed 12 September 2023.

Authors	1	2	3	4	5	6	7	8	9
Nowak et al. [27]	1	1	1	1	0	1	1	1	1
Holsinger et al. [42]	1	1	1	1	1	NR	1	1	1
Tickle et al. [28]	1	1	1	0	NR	1	1	1	1
Buckingham & John [29]	1	1	1	1	0	NR	1	1	1
Olegário et al. [43]	1	1	1	1	NR	1	1	1	1
Tonmukayakul & Arrow [30]	1	NR	NR	NR	NR	1	1	1	1
BaniHani et al. [31]	1	1	1	1	1	1	1	NR	1
Bottega et al. [32]	1	1	1	1	1	1	1	1	1
Schwendicke et al. [43]	1	1	NR	NR	NR	1	1	1	1
de Moura et al. [46]	1	1	1	1	1	1	0	1	1
Elamin et al. [45]	1	1	1	1	1	NR	1	1	1
Schwendicke et al. [47]	1	1	1	NA	NR	1	0	1	1
Davis et al. [33]	1	1	NA	1	1	1	1	1	1

Table 3. Cont.

Authors	1	2	3	4	5	6	7	8	9	10	11	12	13	14	Total	Grading	Quality Assessment
Homer et al. [34]	1	1	0	NR	NR	1	0	1	1	0	1	NR	1	1	11	Good	For observational and cross-sectional studies
Maguire et al. [49]	1	1	0	0	0	1	0	1	1	0	1	NR	0	1	10	Fair	For observational and cross-sectional studies
Nowak et al. [27]	1	1	1	1	0	1	1	1	1	NR	1	1	1	1	11	Good	For controlled intervention studies
Olegário et al. [48]	1	1	1	1	NR	1	1	1	1	1	1	0	1	0	10	Fair	For observational and cross-sectional studies
Zaror et al. [18]	1	1	1	1	1	1	NR	NR	1	1	1	1	1	1	13	Good	For controlled intervention studies
Effenberger et al. [38]	1	1	0	0	1	1	0	0	1	1	1	0	1	1	9	Fair	For controlled intervention studies
Elhennawy et al. [36]	1	1	0	0	1	1	1	1	1	1	1	0	1	0	11	Good	For observational and cross-sectional studies
Halasa-Rappel et al. [37]	1	1	1	1	1	0	1	1	1	1	1	0	1	1	13	Good	For controlled intervention studies
Nantanee & Sriratanaban [41]	1	1	1	1	0	1	1	1	1								
Nguyen et al. [39]	1	1	1	1	0	1	NA	NA	1								
Aly et al. [40]	1	1	0	0	1	1	1	1	1								

Legend: NA (not applicable); CD (cannot determine); NR (not reported)

Grading for CCSS: 0–5 = poor; 6–10 = fair; 11–14 = good

Grading for CIS: 0–5 = poor; 6–10 = fair; 11–14 = good

Table 3. Cont.

Authors	1	2	3	4	5	6	7	8	9
1	1	1	1	11	Good		For controlled intervention studies		
1	1	1	1	13	Good		For controlled intervention studies		
1	1	1	0	12	Good		For controlled intervention studies		
1	1	1	1	11	Good		For controlled intervention studies		
0	0	NA	1	10	Fair		For observational and cross-sectional studies		
1	0	1	1	9	Fair		For controlled intervention studies		
1	1	1	1	10	Fair		For controlled intervention studies		
1	1	1	1	13	Good		For controlled intervention studies		
1	1	1	1	13	Good		For controlled intervention studies		
1	0	1	0	10	Fair		For controlled intervention studies		
1	0	1	0	8	Fair		For controlled intervention studies		
1	0	1	1	11	Good		For controlled intervention studies		
0	NA	NR	1	10	Fair		For observational and cross-sectional studies		
1	1	0	0	11	Good		For observational and cross-sectional studies		
0	0	NR	0	7	Fair		For observational and cross-sectional studies		
1	1	1	1	11	Good		For controlled intervention studies		

Table 4. Studies included in the systematic review with information on ID no., authors, year of publication, source of publication, place of study conduct, cost of treatment (intervention), cost of control group, and clinical outcome.

II	Authors	Year	Country	Treatment Costs	Control Costs	Clinical Results
				Prevention		
				Education		
1	Nowak et al. [27]	2014	USA	Early starters: fillings USD 3.11 ± 3.77, crowns 2.28 ± 3.35, pulpotomies USD 1.57 ± 2.66, extractions USD 0.72 ± 1.44, total 7.69 ± 8.61 USD/child/treatment	Late starters: fillings USD 3.96 ± 5.09, crowns USD 3.47 ± 5.13, pulpotomies USD 2.42 ± 4.27, extractions USD 1.41 ± 2.72, total 11.27 ± 12.56 USD/child/treatment	1. Early starters received fewer treatments for restorations, crowns, pulpotomies, and extractions than late starters. 2. Early starters had lower expenditures for treatment procedures than late starters
				Sealing		
2	Halasa-Rappel et al. [37]	2021	USA	Pit-and-fissure sealing: 75 USD/molar	No pit-and-fissure sealing: 90 USD/molar	Pit-and-fissure sealing of healthy molars in high-risk children would save USD 25 per molar and result in an additional caries-free molar year over a 5-year follow-up period
				Fluoride varnish		
3	Zaror et al. [18]	2020	Chile	Fluoride varnish: 98.76 CLP/child	Control: 98.74 CLP/child	The fluoride varnish protocol is more effective and less expensive in preventing ECC in non-fluoridated areas
4	McMahon et al. [35]	2020	UK	Fluoride varnish plus treatment as usual (TAU) Childsmile program interventions: 32.66 (SD 13.21) GBP/child	TAU Childsmile interventions (Cost: N/A)	An NNT of 21 and cost of GBP 686 to prevent a single worsening of d3mft were calculated. FV is unlikely to be an effective or cost-effective addition to the program
5	Buckingham & John [29]	2017	UK	Fluoride varnish applications (one, two, and three): 71 GBP/child, 88 GBP/child/2 yr	No control	Establishing community fluoride varnish programs requires significant investment, and the long-term benefits in practice are unclear. In addition to fluoridation, dietary improvement is needed to reduce the extent of caries

Table 4. Cont.

II	Authors	Year	Country	Treatment Costs	Control Costs	Clinical Results
6	Tickle et al. [28]	2016	UK	The intervention was composite in nature and included a varnish containing 22,600 parts per million (ppm) fluoride, a toothbrush, and a 50-mL tube of toothpaste containing 1450 ppm fluoride; and standardized, evidence-based prevention counseling at semiannual intervals for 3 years: 155.74 GBP/child	The control group received prevention counseling alone: 48.21 GBP/child	No statistically significant effect could be demonstrated for the primary endpoint. Once caries develops, pain is to be expected. There was a statistically significant difference in dmfs in caries-active children in favor of the intervention. Although the intervention was sufficiently effective, the impact was small and the clinical and economic benefits were questionable
7	Homer et al. [34]	2020	UK	Conventional with best practice prevention (C + P), C + P (e.g., local anesthesia, removal of carious tissue and restoration): 250.48 (221.70) GBP/child	Biological with best practice prevention (B + P; e.g., partial/no removal and restoration of carious tissue): 231.28 (214.47) GBP/child, or best practice prevention alone (PA): 211.32 (257.28) GBP/child	At the thresholds (mean cost), B + P has the highest probability of being considered cost-effective. Beyond the willingness-to-pay thresholds considered, the probability of B + P being considered cost-effective never exceeded 75%
8	Maguire et al. [49]	2020	UK	(1) Best practice prevention (local anesthesia, removal of carious tissue, placement of fillings): 250.48 (221.70) GBP/child	(2) Best practice prevention (sealing of caries, selective removal of carious tissue, and fissure sealing): 231.28 (214.47) GBP/child, and (3) best practice prevention alone (dietary and toothbrushing counseling, topical fluoride, and fissure sealing) of permanent teeth: 211.32 (257.28) GBP/child	There was no evidence of an overall difference between the three treatment approaches in the incidence or number of episodes of toothache or infection or both, during the follow-up period
9	Effenberger et al. [38]	2022	South Africa	Fluoride varnish every 3 months and supervised brushing with fluoridated toothpaste: 1667 (SD 1055) ZAR/child	No fluoride varnish, supervised tooth brushing with fluoridated toothpaste: ZAR 950 (SD 943)	Regular application of fluoride varnish in addition to daily tooth brushing under supervision had no significant caries preventive effect and was not cost-effective
10	Nantanee & Sriratanaban [41]	2023	Thailand	Fluoride varnish: 50.30 ± 24.14 THB per visit/child	No control	The fluoride varnish application program in one to three sessions during visits in healthy children appears to be cost-effective and shows estimated net benefits of interventions to prevent dental caries. These results suggest that children between the ages of 9 and 30 months should have at least three visits of the fluoride varnish application program during child care visits

Table 4. Cont.

Authors	Year	Country	Treatment Costs	Control Costs	Clinical Results
			Silver diamine fluoride (SDF) and atraumatic restorative treatment (ART)		
11 Nguyen et al. [39]	2022	Australia	Children receiving SDF + standard care: AUD 409.90 (SD 36.24); SDF protocol intervention: AUD 3.48 per child	Children receiving SDF—no standard care; SDF protocol intervention: AUD 3.48 per child	The SDF protocol intervention is a cost-effective option for the treatment of dental caries in young children
12 Tonmukayakul & Arrow [30]	2017	Australia	Atraumatic restorative treatment (ART): AUD 1085.51 (includes general anesthesia (GA))	Standard care (SC): AUD 1403.28 (incl. GA)	Children in the ART-based group received more dental services than those in the SC group. The ART-based approach appears to be a worthwhile intervention, as it resulted in fewer referred cases and allowed more treatments to be delivered with cost savings
13 Bottega et al. [32]	2018	Brazil	Papacarie group (caries removal with the chemical-mechanical method—Papacarie gel): 0.91 BRL/procedure	Drill group (caries removal with the traditional method—drilling): 1.37 BRL/procedure	Papacarie offers an excellent cost advantage for minimally invasive removal of carious tissue and is a viable alternative for public health care
14 Aly et al. [40]	2023	Egypt	Silver-modified atraumatic restorative treatment (SMART): 67 EGP (USD 2.17)/average cost per restoration of the two study arms	Atraumatic restorative treatment (ART): 61 EGP (USD 1.97)/average cost per restoration of the two study arms	The use of SMART technology could change paradigms in caries management. Because it is a patient-friendly and cost-effective approach, it could be used as a superior treatment option in treating young children, people with behavioral and medical problems, and to promote access to oral care for the disadvantaged
15 Davis et al. [33]	2020	USA	Silver diamine fluoride (SDF): 619.72 USD (SD 563.51)/child/year (number of visits/dental treatments and expenditures)	No SDF: 958.04 USD (SD 824.65)/child/year (number of visits/dental treatments and expenditures)	SDF can result in cost savings when used as an adjunct to, rather than a complete replacement for, restorative treatment in young children
16 BaniHani et al. [31]	2018	UK	Non-selective removal of hard dentin with/without pulp therapy: 168.68 GBP/child	Selective removal of solid dentin and Hall technique: 78.97 GBP/child	Although both approaches achieved similar successful results, the biological approach, which consisted mainly of the Hall technique, was associated with lower treatment costs. Both approaches were positively received by the children and caregivers

Table 4. *Cont.*

ID	Authors	Year	Country	Treatment Costs	Control Costs	Clinical Results
17	Elhennawy et al. [36]	2021	Germany	Selective caries removal (SE): 68.4 EUR (20.1) (initial cost)/1 molar/child; total treatment cost after 24 months: EUR 85 (74); total cost after 24 months: EUR 106 (90)	Stepwise caries removal (SW): 132.9 EUR (18.3) (initial cost)/1 molar/child; total treatment cost after 24 months: EUR 141 (44); total cost after 24 months: EUR 176 (51)	In deciduous molars with clearly defined deep carious lesions, SE was less expensive and similarly effective to SW. For cost and applicability reasons, SW may have to be indicated restrictively, e.g., only for very deep lesions (>3/4 dentin extension)
				Restoration		
				Filling		
18	de Moura et al. [46]	2019	Brazil	Vitro Molar®: low-cost GIC (exact cost: N/A)	Ketac Molar®: high-viscosity GIC (exact cost: N/A)	The success rate for restorations with low-cost GIC (Vitro Molar®) was particularly high after six months. However, one year later, restorations performed with high-viscosity GIC (Ketac Molar®) in primary second molars with small or medium cavities were more successful than those indicated for ART with low-cost GIC
19	Olegário et al. [43]	2017	Brazil	G1-GC Fuji IX Gold Label 9 (GC Corp): 55 BRL/package	G2-Vitro Molar (DFL): 25 BRL/package and G3-Maxxion R (FGM): 9.4 BRL/package.	The low-cost GICs perform worse than GC Fuji Gold Label 9 in occlusal ART restorations in deciduous molars
20	Olegário et al. [48]	2020	Brazil	G1-GC Fuji IX Gold Label 9 (GC Corp): BRL 4.66 (0.13) (baseline); BRL 5.32 (0.28); BRL 5.88 (0.38) (2-year total cost).	G2-Vitro Molar (DFL): BRL 3.65 (0.11) (baseline); BRL 5.225 (0.30) (2-year total cost) and G3-Maxxion R (FGM): BRL 3.37 (0.08) (baseline); BRL 4.84 (0.26) (2-year total cost)	The use of GC Gold Label 9 shows a higher survival rate compared to Maxxion R and Vitro Molar for occlusal ART restorations in primary molars, i.e., low-cost GICs perform worse than GC Gold Label 9 for occlusal ART restorations in primary molars
				Crown		
21	Schwendicke et al. [44]	2018	Germany	Hall technique (HT): 66 (62–71) EUR/child (1 molar)	Non-restorative cavity control (NRCC): 296 (274–318) EUR/child (1 molar) and conventional removal and restoration of carious tissue (CR): 83 (73–92) EUR/child (1 molar)	HT was more cost-effective than CR or NRCC in treating cavitated caries lesions in deciduous molars and resulted in better dental health outcomes at lower cost

Table 4. Cont.

ID	Authors	Year	Country	Treatment Costs	Control Costs	Clinical Results
22	Elamin et al. [45]	2019	Sudan	Preformed metal crowns (PMCs) placed using conventional techniques (CT): 7.81 SDG/unit	PMCs placed by biological reverberation techniques (HT): 2.45 SDG/unit	PMCs placed using the Hall technique or conventional techniques have excellent survival rates in disadvantaged communities. Extremely cost-effective in terms of materials, labor, and time, HT is a successful and cost-effective public health intervention for carious deciduous molars in communities and developing countries
23	Schwendicke et al. [47]	2019	UK	Hall technique (HT)—intervention: 24 (23–25) GBP/child/molar (base case analysis); 32.26 (30.83–33.98) GBP/child/molar	Conventional removal and restoration of carious tissue (CR): 29 (25–34) GBP/child/molar (base case analysis); 48.91 (34.40–68.74) GBP/child/molar	Based on a long-term practice-based study, HT was more cost-effective than CR because HT was maintained longer and fewer complications occurred at a lower cost
24	Holsinger et al. [42]	2016	USA	Zircon crowns; zircon crown: USD 23.48 (approximate cost of crown mold), USD 28.38 (total estimated cost of materials/treatment)	No control—cost indicated for: resin-veneered stainless-steel crown: USD 18.70 (approximate crown mold cost), USD 24.13 (estimated total material/treatment cost); strip crown: USD 6.18 (approximate crown mold cost), USD 21.83 (estimated total material/treatment cost)	Zirconia crowns are clinically acceptable restorations in the primary maxillary anterior dentition

4. Discussion

4.1. Aim of the Study and Main Findings

The aim of this study was to systematically review and summarize current research on the cost-effectiveness of treatment decisions for early childhood caries (ECC) in infants and toddlers. Using ad hoc search terms (MeSH), keywords, and a defined search strategy, the electronic databases Scopus, MEDLINE via PubMed, Embase, and gray literature were searched. Observational epidemiologic studies, i.e., cohort studies, case–control studies, and randomized controlled trials that reported on the cost-effectiveness of treatment decisions of early childhood caries in infants and toddlers, according to the PRISMA guidelines, were included in the study. Cost-effectiveness modeling (e.g., Markov model) or cost simulation without direct link to clinical intervention were explicitly excluded. This systematic review is one of the very few systematic reviews focusing on cost-effectiveness in children [50]. However, to the best of our knowledge, no systematic review of treatment decisions for ECC in infants and toddlers has been conducted so far. A total of 494 articles were identified, and after title and abstract evaluation, hand searching, and full-text review, 24 full-text articles were finally included in the systematic review [12,20–42], with 17 articles classified as prevention [18,27–41,49] and seven articles classified as restoration [35–41]. Dental caries remains the most common disease in humans [51,52], and early childhood caries in infants and toddlers from birth to approximately age seven can have serious health and economic consequences [2,3,9]. Non-treatment can lead to serious infections, developmental disorders, and massive losses in quality of life as well as financial burdens [8,9,15]. Depending on the severity, treatment is often only possible with sedation measures or even general anesthesia [8,16].

4.2. Classification of Studies

Although the included studies could be classified/assigned into the two areas of prevention and restoration [18,27–49], each with subgroups on (1) prevention: education/outreach, sealing, fluoride varnish, and silver diamine fluoride (SDF) and atraumatic restorative treatment (ART) [18,27–41,49] and on (2) restoration with filling and crown restoration [35–41], a concrete comparison was very difficult due to the lack of homogeneity in the results. Direct comparisons between the groups could be drawn neither related to the therapeutic intervention nor to the methodology used to measure cost-effectiveness. However, due to the given heterogeneity in the results, neither a further synthesis nor a meta-analysis could be performed. In addition to the limitation that the systematic review included too few studies or that no more literature was available in the electronic databases without a time limit, the prevailing socioeconomic, cultural, and ethnic backgrounds in the respective country or state must be considered for comparison or evaluation of the treatment methods and cost-effectiveness.

4.3. Geographical and Substantive Differences

While most studies have been conducted in the United Kingdom of Great Britain and Northern Ireland, the public health system in the countries of England, Wales, Scotland, and Northern Ireland must be considered for population care [28,29,31,34,35,47,49]. In direct comparison to the United States (USA) [27,33,37,42], unlike the United Kingdom of Great Britain and Northern Ireland, the USA does not have direct universal coverage or government health protection through health insurance for the entire population. This is in clear contrast to the German health care system [36,43], which finances dental care or oral health care through the German social insurance system in addition to accident, pension, unemployment, and long-term care insurance in the statutory health insurance as well as the private health insurance or guarantees health care including oral health and teeth for the legally insured [36,43]. Accordingly, there is a statutory legal entitlement to comprehensive care with services that are sufficient, appropriate, and economical and do not exceed what is necessary. Although similar, the same conditions are not offered to permanent residents in Australia, so that while medical services are fully subsidized, dental services are only partially subsidized by government insurance [30,39]. To be able to make valid statements about the oral health care, the prevention and restoration measures for ECC in the respective countries, the gross national product (GNP), the care options (type of practices, comprehensive or patchy care), the health protection (health insurance), if existing, individual and group prophylaxis programs (public health care), as well as the access to oral health care would have to be examined when taking the cost-effectiveness into account.

Only one study each on outreach/education/education [27] and sealing [37] were identified; however, the findings are not comparable. The data on pitting and fissure sealing in healthy molars in children at high risk of caries would save approximately USD 25 with a documented follow-up period of five years in the USA [37]. Unfortunately, these data are not comparable due to a lack of evidence, and the statement is therefore not very meaningful regarding cost-effectiveness.

However, regarding the first visit to the dentist, one study was conducted in a large number of children, also in the USA [27], showing that children treated by a dentist for the first time below the age of four years required fewer treatments such as restorations, crowns, pulpotomies, or extractions than children treated by a dentist for the first time when they were over four years old [27]. This fact can also be observed by dentists in individual and group prophylaxis programs in Germany [15]. Lower expenditure demonstrates the cost-effectiveness of getting children used to the dentist and oral care measures as a part of daily personal hygiene at an early age. Additionally, it is encouraging that nowadays in Central European countries, primary prophylaxis is increasingly performed routinely, often in an interdisciplinary way by gynecologists and midwives in cooperation with dentists [15]. In this program, mothers-to-be are already informed and educated about various topics such as sugar consumption and nutrition, oral hygiene, and dental care for their future infants and toddlers [15]. Pre-school prophylaxis then includes prophylaxis at the dentist's office and in kindergarten through visits by the health department or dentists. The daily habits of brushing teeth with fluoride toothpaste and toothbrush from the first tooth and the regular application of fluoride varnish at the dentist's visit are introduced at these times and often practiced through play and reward systems [15].

Unfortunately, the different types of treatments reported in the included studies do not allow for a more detailed, concrete assessment of cost-effectiveness, such as with fluoride varnish; although randomized controlled trials have been conducted [18,28,35,36,38,41,49], the statements provide little meaningful results with fluoride varnish application at 98.76 CLP/child in Chile [18] but at 155.74 GBP/child or a combination of prevention and restoration at 250 GBP/child [34,49] in the United Kingdom of Great Britain and Northern Ireland [28]. Although on one hand, in Chile, the fluoride varnish protocol is reported to be more effective and cost-effective in preventing early childhood caries, contradictory results are reported in the United Kingdom of Great Britain and Northern Ireland, such that fluoride varnish application is sufficiently effective, but the effect is only small and the clinical and economic benefits are even questionable [28]. Other studies even documented no difference between the different treatment approaches in terms of clinical outcome [33,49]. No differences in the occurrence or number of toothache episodes or infections due to early carious lesions were also observed over the observation period when comparing the intervention group with the control group, with cost effectiveness slightly in the direction of fluoride varnish application [33,49].

On one hand, it is highly questionable when, based on uncontrolled studies, statements are made that the application of fluoride varnish in one to three sessions in healthy children appears to be cost-effective and therefore the estimated benefit for the prevention of early childhood caries is given [41]. On the other hand, contradictory statements on regular fluoride varnish application in addition to daily tooth brushing under guardian supervision were reported without significant caries preventive effect and even without cost-effectiveness in a study from South Africa [38].

4.4. Limitations

This systematic review has several limitations. There is a lack of current prevalence data on the experience of ECC in infants and toddlers and cost-effectiveness studies in numerous countries worldwide. While there are many publications from the United Kingdom of Great Britain and Northern Ireland [28,29,31,33,35,47,49], the United States [27,33,37,42], and Brazil with low to moderate number of publications [32,43,46,48], in the American continent, nine studies [18,27,32,33,37,42,43,46,48]; in the African continent, three studies [38,41,45]; in the Australian continent, two studies [30,39]; and in the Asian continent, only one study [41] were available. In addition to the data on cost-effectiveness in ECC in infants and toddlers from the United Kingdom of Great Britain and Northern Ireland, few relevant data were available in the literature meeting the search criteria of the study to be included in the study. However, because the two continents of Europe and the Americas are reasonably well distributed across the globe, they can at least provide a general estimate of the prevalence of ECC and the importance of cost-effectiveness in this geographic area. It should also be remembered that health data are not generally collected or available for all countries worldwide, clearly affecting the overall estimate of global prevalence. Because the data in the studies were collected in regional or local populations, the results may be only partially representative of the overall situation at the country level. Relatively few studies overall could be included in the systematic review. Although data collection worldwide on cost-effectiveness in public health was initiated in many places about a decade ago, the information is still not extensive and therefore limited. This also means that the statements so far are of little to no significance regarding various preventive as well as restorative therapeutic decision-making processes. The accuracy of the collected and summarized data is also directly dependent on the accuracy of the included data and should therefore be interpreted with caution. Generalization of the data to the respective preventive and restorative therapeutic decisions studied should be made very cautiously, or even avoided, according to the current assessment of the evidence regarding clinical outcomes in cost-effectiveness studies, until the knowledge gaps in the literature are closed.

However, the included studies might show that the prevalence of ECC in infants and toddlers varies widely across geographic areas. More research is needed to monitor oral health status at the individual level (parents or guardians and children), as there is a clear link between healthy oral habits and socioeconomic challenges within societies. This underscores the need for further research on socioeconomic indicators related to socioeconomic, cultural, and ethnic disparities, regardless of the target projection to minority or vulnerable populations. The problem of persistently high caries prevalence can be solved by addressing the needs of parents or guardians in the community with full consideration of the socioeconomic, cultural, as well as ethnic backgrounds. The success of ECC prevention programs depends directly on parents and guardians, but also on doctors and dentists. They are responsible for educating and protecting general and oral health of infants and toddlers. These prevention programs for ECC must be developed with a clear understanding of the individual needs of society and its socioeconomic, cultural, and ethnic circumstances with all decision-makers involved in the health process. Only in this way, will it be possible, together with all decision-makers, to make better treatment decisions in the future, in the sense of a best-practice approach or from a health, economic, and political point of view. Spread of ECC in infants and toddlers must be prevented to avoid the serious consequences of incorrect or inadequate oral and dental hygiene, such as possible damage to the germs of permanent teeth, impaired tooth eruption, developmental disorders of the upper and lower jaws, impaired speech development, insufficient nutritional behavior, dysfunctional chewing, and swallowing ability, but also psychosocial problems. The goal must also be to prevent chewing and swallowing disorders, as well as psychosocial developmental deficits and lack of compliance in future dental visits due to early caries experience.

5. Conclusions

The enormously important aspect of public health care 'cost-effectiveness' was systematically examined in this study in relation to treatment decisions for ECC in infants and young children, and the following conclusions can be drawn within the limitations of the present study:

1. Statements on the cost-effectiveness of individual therapeutic interventions in the fields of prevention and restoration are difficult due to the heterogeneity in the results or the different methodologies used in the studies included.
2. Despite numerous randomized controlled clinical trials with follow-up periods of often 24 months, the efficacy of individual interventions is sometimes contradictory in terms of clinical outcome.
3. Socioeconomic, cultural, and ethnic differences must be considered when comparing conditions in terms of cost-effectiveness.
4. Studies on cost-effectiveness of therapeutic treatment decisions for early childhood caries have been conducted for about ten years; since then, the number has increased significantly.
5. An important paradigm shift can be observed, away from surgical/restorative approaches and toward increased therapeutic/medical intervention with a focus on prevention.

Supplementary Materials: The following supporting information can be downloaded at: https://www.mdpi.com/article/10.3390/medicina59101865/s1, Figure S1: PRISMA 2020 checklist; Table S1: Excluded studies; Figure S2: PRISMA flow diagram.

Author Contributions: Conceptualization, T.G.W.; methodology, T.G.W. and G.C.; software, T.G.W.; validation, T.G.W. and G.C.; formal analysis, T.G.W.; investigation, T.G.W.; resources, T.G.W.; data curation, T.G.W. and G.C.; writing—original draft preparation, T.G.W.; writing—review and editing, T.G.W. and G.C.; project administration, T.G.W. All authors have read and agreed to the published version of the manuscript.

Funding: This research received no external funding.

Institutional Review Board Statement: Not applicable.

Informed Consent Statement: Not applicable.

Data Availability Statement: Data sharing is not applicable to this article as no new data were created or analyzed in this study.

Acknowledgments: This systematic review paper was partially T.G.W.'s master's thesis in the distance learning program "Management of Health and Social Care Institutions" approved by the scientific management and the examination board of the Distance and Independent Studies Center (DISC) of the University of Kaiserslautern-Landau (RPTU) (formerly Technical University (TU) Kaiserslautern), indicated and recommended for publication.

Conflicts of Interest: The authors declare no conflict of interest.

References

1. Wyne, A.H. Early childhood caries: Nomenclature and case definition. *Community Dent. Oral Epidemiol.* **1999**, *27*, 313–315. [CrossRef]
2. Colak, H.; Dülgergil, C.T.; Dalli, M.; Hamidi, M.M. Early childhood caries update: A review of causes, diagnoses, and treatments. *J. Nat. Sci. Biol. Med.* **2013**, *4*, 29–38.
3. Seow, W.K. Biological mechanisms of early childhood caries. *Community Dent. Oral Epidemiol.* **1998**, *26* (Suppl. 1), 8–27. [CrossRef]
4. Ramos-Gomez, F.J.; Weintraub, J.A.; Gansky, S.A.; Hoover, C.I.; Featherstone, J.D.B. Bacterial, behavioral and environmental factors associated with early childhood caries. *J. Clin. Pediatr. Dent.* **2002**, *26*, 165–173. [CrossRef]
5. Anil, S.; Anand, P.S. Early Childhood Caries: Prevalence, risk factors, and prevention. *Front. Pediatr.* **2017**, *5*, 157. [CrossRef]
6. Pitts, N.B.; Zero, D.T.; Marsh, P.D.; Ekstrand, K.; Weintraub, J.A.; Ramos-Gomez, F.; Tagami, J.; Twetman, S.; Tsakos, G.; Ismail, A. Dental caries. *Nat. Rev. Dis. Primers* **2017**, *3*, 17030. [CrossRef]

7. American Academy of Pediatric Dentistry. Policy on early childhood caries (ECC): Classifications, consequences, and preventive strategies. In *The Reference Manual of Pediatric Dentistry*; American Academy of Pediatric Dentistry: Chicago, IL, USA, 2020; pp. 79–81.
8. Robke, F.J. Consequences of teat bottle abuse for dental health. Prevalence of caries, dental and jaw malocclusions in northern German preschool children. *J. Orofac.* **2008**, *69*, 5–19. [CrossRef]
9. Splieth, C.; Treuner, A.; Berndt, C. Oral health in young children. *Prev. Health Issues* **2009**, *4*, 119–123.
10. Hippke, A. Caries in one and two year old daycare center children in Hamburg. *Dissertation*. 2012. Available online: https://ediss.sub.uni-hamburg.de/bitstream/ediss/4958/1/Dissertation.pdf (accessed on 13 October 2023).
11. Borutta, A.; Wagner, M.; Kneist, S. Condition structure of early childhood caries. *Oral Prophyl. Ped Dent.* **2010**, *32*, 58–63.
12. Treuner, A.; Splieth, C. Early childhood caries-facts and prevention. *Dent Communic.* **2013**, *17*, 44–50.
13. Rojas, G.; Deichsel, M.; Lüdecke, K.; Heinrich-Weltzien, R. Results of a Nationwide Study in the State of Brandenburg. Available online: www.Brandenburger-kinderzaehne.de/Veroeffentlichungen294.0.html (accessed on 12 September 2023).
14. Robke, F.J.; Buitkamp, M. Incidence of teat bottle caries in preschool children in a West German city. *Oral Prophyl.* **2002**, *24*, 59–65.
15. Kassenzahnärztliche Bundesvereinigung (KZBV), Bundeszahnärztekammer (BZÄK). Preventing Early Childhood Caries—A Concept for Dental Prevention in Young Children. Available online: https://www.kzbv.de/fruehkindliche-karies-vermeiden.1030.de.html (accessed on 12 September 2023).
16. Lee, H.H.; Milgrom, P.; Starks, H.; Burke, W. Trends in death associated with pediatric dental sedation and general anesthesia. *Paediatr. Anaesth.* **2013**, *23*, 741–746. [CrossRef]
17. Heinen, N. Death at the Pediatric Dentist. Available online: https://www.welt.de/wissenschaft/plus245125756/Tod-beim-Kinderzahnarzt-Gefaehrliche-Narkosen-Wenn-Kinder-im-Zahnarztstuhl-sterben.html (accessed on 12 September 2023).
18. Zaror, C.; Muñoz-Millàn, P.; Espinoza-Espinoza, G.; Vergara-Gonzàlez, C.; Martìnez-Zapata, M.J. Cost-effectiveness of adding fluoride varnish to a preventive protocol for early childhood caries in rural children with no access to fluoridated drinking water. *J. Dent.* **2020**, *98*, 103374. [CrossRef]
19. Tonmukayakul, U.; Forrest, H.; Arrow, P. Cost-effectiveness analysis of atraumatic restorative treatment to manage early childhood caries: Microsimulation modeling. *Aust. Dent. J.* **2021**, *66*, S63–S70. [CrossRef]
20. Rodriguez, G.A.; Cabello, R.A.; Borroni, C.P.; Palacio, R.A. Cost-effectiveness of probiotics and fluoride varnish in caries prevention in preschool children. *J. Public Health Dent.* **2002**, *82*, 280–288. [CrossRef]
21. Centers for Disease Control and Prevention. Cost-Effectiveness Analysis (2023). Available online: https://www.cdc.gov/policy/polaris/economics/cost-effectiveness/index.html (accessed on 13 October 2023).
22. Wolf, T. Cost-Effectiveness of Treatment Decisions for Early Childhood Caries in Infants and Young Children. Open Science Framework (OSF). Available online: osf.io/cmw58 (accessed on 12 September 2023).
23. Page, M.J.; McKenzie, J.E.; Bossuyt, P.M.; Boutron, I.; Hoffmann, T.C.; Mulrow, C.D.; Shamseer, L.; Tetzlaff, J.M.; Akl, E.A.; Brennan, S.E.; et al. The PRISMA 2020 statement: An updated guideline for reporting systematic reviews. *BMJ* **2021**, *372*, n71. [CrossRef]
24. Santos, C.M.C.; Pimenta, C.A.M.; Nobre, M.R.C. The PICO strategy for the research question construction and evidence search. *Rev. Lat. Am. Enferm.* **2007**, *14*, 508–511. [CrossRef]
25. Cooke, A.; Smith, D.; Booth, A. Beyond PICO: The SPIDER tool for qualitative evidence synthesis. *Qual. Health Res.* **2012**, *22*, 1435–1443. [CrossRef]
26. Methley, A.M.; Campbell, S.; Chew-Graham, C.; McNally, R.; Cheraghi-Sohi, S. PICO, PICOS and SPIDER: A comparison study of specificity and sensitivity in three search tools for qualitative systematic reviews. *BMC Health Serv. Res.* **2014**, *14*, 579. [CrossRef]
27. Nowak, A.J.; Casamassimo, P.S.; Scott, J.; Moulton, R. Do early dental visits reduce treatment and treatment costs for children? *Pediatr. Dent.* **2014**, *36*, 489–493.
28. Tickle, M.; O'Neill, C.; Donaldson, M.; Birch, S.; Noble, S.; Killough, S.; Murphy, L.; Greer, M.; Brodison, J.; Verghis, R.; et al. A randomised controlled trial to measure the effects and costs of a dental caries prevention regime for young children attending primary care dental services: The Northern Ireland Caries Prevention in Practice NIC-PIP trial. *Health Technol. Assess.* **2016**, *20*, 1–96. [CrossRef]
29. Buckingham, S.; John, J.H. Outcomes and costs of pre-school and school-based fluoride varnish pilots. *Br. Dent. J.* **2017**, *222*, 591–594. [CrossRef]
30. Tonmukayakul, U.; Arrow, P. Cost-effectiveness analysis of the atraumatic restorative treatment-based approach to managing early childhood caries. *Community Dent. Oral Epidemiol.* **2017**, *45*, 92–100. [CrossRef]
31. BaniHani, A.; Deery, C.; Toumba, J.; Duggal, M. Effectiveness, costs and patient acceptance of a conventional and a biological treatment approach for carious primary teeth in children. *Caries Res.* **2019**, *53*, 65–75. [CrossRef]
32. Bottega, F.; Bussadori, S.K.; Endruweit Battisti, I.D.; Paveglio Vieria, E.; Szambelan Pompeo, T.; Winkelmann, E.F. Costs and benefits of Papacarie in pediatric dentistry: A randomized clinical trial. *Sci. Rep.* **2018**, *8*, 17908. [CrossRef]
33. Davis, M.R.; Johnson, E.L.; Meyer, B.D. Comparing dental treatment between children receiving and not receiving Silver Diamine Fluoride. *J. Clin. Pediatr. Dent.* **2020**, *44*, 400–406. [CrossRef]
34. Homer, T.; Maguire, A.; Douglas, G.V.A.; Innes, N.P.; Clarkson, J.E.; Wilson, N.; Ryan, V.; McColl, E.; Robertson, M.; Vale, L. Cost-effectiveness of child caries management: A randomised controlled trial (FiCTION trial). *BMC Oral Health* **2021**, *20*, 45. [CrossRef]

35. McMahon, A.D.; Wright, W.; Anopa, Y.; McIntosh, E.; Turner, S.; Conway, D.I.; Macpherson, L.M.D. Fluoride varnish in nursery schools: A randomised controlled trial–Protecting teeth @3. *Caries Res.* **2020**, *54*, 274–282. [CrossRef]
36. Elhennawy, K.; Finke, C.; Paris, S.; Reda, S.; Jost-Brinkmann, P.G.; Schwendicke, F. Selective vs. stepwise removal of deep carious lesions in primary molars: 24 months follow-up from a randomized controlled trial. *Clin. Oral Investig.* **2021**, *25*, 645–652. [CrossRef]
37. Halasa-Rappel, Y.; Archibald, J.; Miller, P.; Frederick Lambert, R.; Hong, M.; Ng, M.W.; Sulyanto, R. Pit-and-fissure sealants on primary molars are a cost savings. *J. Am. Dent. Assoc.* **2021**, *152*, 832–841. [CrossRef]
38. Effenberger, S.; Greenwall, L.; Cebula, M.; Myburgh, N.; Simpson, K.; Smit, D.; Wicht, M.J.; Schwendicke, F. Cost-effectiveness and efficacy of fluoride varnish for caries prevention in South African children: A cluster-randomized controlled community trial. *Community Dent. Oral Epidemiol.* **2022**, *50*, 453–460. [CrossRef]
39. Nguyen, T.M.; Tonmukayakul, U.; Hall, M.; Calache, H. Cost-effectiveness analysis of silver diamine fluoride to divert dental general anaesthesia compared to standard care. *Aust. Dent. J.* **2022**, *67*, 352–361. [CrossRef]
40. Aly, A.A.M.; Aziz, A.M.A.; Elghazawy, R.K.; El Fald, R.K.A. Survival analysis and cost effectiveness of Silver Modified Atraumatic Restorative Treatment SMART and ART occlusal restorations in primary molars: A randomized controlled trial. *J. Dent.* **2023**, *128*, 104379. [CrossRef]
41. Nantanee, R.; Sriratanaban, J. Cost-effectiveness and estimated net monetary benefits of a fluoride varnish application program during well-child visits by 9- to 30-month-old children in three areas of Thailand. *Community Dent. Oral Epidemiol.* **2023**, *51*, 512–518. [CrossRef]
42. Holsinger, D.M.; Wells, M.H.; Scarbecz, M.; Donaldson, M. Clinical evaluation and parental satisfaction with pediatric zirconia anterior crowns. *Pediatr. Dent.* **2016**, *38*, 192–197.
43. Olegário, I.C.; de Brito Pacheco, A.L.; de Araujo, M.P.; de Miranda Ladewig, N.; Calil Bonifacio, C.; Pettorosi Imparato, J.C.; Procida Raggio, D. Low-cost GICs reduce survival rate in occlusal ART restorations in primary molars after one year: A RCT. *J. Dent.* **2017**, *57*, 45–50. [CrossRef]
44. Schwendicke, F.; Krois, J.; Splieth, C.H.; Innes, N.; Robertson, M.; Schmöckel, J.; Santamaria, R.M. Cost-effectiveness of managing cavitated primary molar caries lesions: A randomized trial in Germany. *J. Dent.* **2018**, *78*, 40–45. [CrossRef]
45. Elamin, F.; Abdelazeem, N.; Salah, I.; Mirghani, Y.; Wong, F. A randomized clinical trial comparing Hall vs. conventional technique in placing preformed metal crowns from Sudan. *PLoS ONE* **2019**, *14*, e0217740. [CrossRef]
46. De Moura, M.S.; Sousa, G.P.; Brito, M.H.S.F.; Silva, M.C.C.; Lima, L.D.M.; Moura, L.F.A.D.; Lima, C.C.B. Does low-cost GIC have the same survival rate as high-viscosity GIC in atraumatic restorative treatments? A RCT. *Braz. Oral Res.* **2020**, *33*, e125. [CrossRef]
47. Schwendicke, F.; Krois, J.; Robertson, M.; Splieth, C.; Santamaria, R.; Innes, N. Cost-effectiveness of the Hall technique in a randomized trial. *J. Dent. Res.* **2019**, *98*, 61–67. [CrossRef]
48. Olegário, I.C.; Ladewig, N.M.; Hesse, D.; Bonifacio, C.C.; Braga, M.M.; Pettorossi Imparato, J.C.; Medeiros Mendes, F.; Procida Raggio, D. Is it worth using low-cost glass ionomer cements for occlusal ART restorations in primary molars? 2-year survival and cost analysis of a Randomized clinical trial. *J. Dent.* **2020**, *101*, 103446. [CrossRef]
49. Maguire, A.; Clarkson, J.E.; Douglas, G.V.A.; Ryan, V.; Homer, T.; Marshman, Z.; McColl, E.; Wilson, N.; Vale, L.; Robertson, M.; et al. Best-practice prevention alone or with conventional or biological caries management for 3- to 7-year-olds: The FiCTION three-arm RCT. *Health Technol. Assess.* **2020**, *24*, 1–174. [CrossRef]
50. Anopa, Y.; Conway, D.I. Exploring the cost-effectiveness of child dental caries prevention programmes. Are we comparing apples and oranges? *Evid. Based Dent.* **2020**, *21*, 5–7. [CrossRef]
51. Wolf, T.G.; Cagetti, M.G.; Fisher, J.M.; Seeberger, G.K.; Campus, G. Non-communicable diseases and oral health: An overview. *Front. Oral Health* **2021**, *2*, 725460. [CrossRef]
52. Kassebaum, N.J.; Bernabé, E.; Dahiya, M.; Bhandari, B.; Murray, C.J.L.; Marcenes, W. Global burden of untreated caries. *J. Dent. Res.* **2015**, *94*, 650–658. [CrossRef]

Disclaimer/Publisher's Note: The statements, opinions and data contained in all publications are solely those of the individual author(s) and contributor(s) and not of MDPI and/or the editor(s). MDPI and/or the editor(s) disclaim responsibility for any injury to people or property resulting from any ideas, methods, instructions or products referred to in the content.

MDPI AG
Grosspeteranlage 5
4052 Basel
Switzerland
Tel.: +41 61 683 77 34

Medicina Editorial Office
E-mail: medicina@mdpi.com
www.mdpi.com/journal/medicina

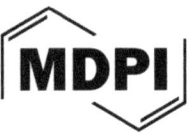

Disclaimer/Publisher's Note: The title and front matter of this reprint are at the discretion of the Guest Editor. The publisher is not responsible for their content or any associated concerns. The statements, opinions and data contained in all individual articles are solely those of the individual Editor and contributors and not of MDPI. MDPI disclaims responsibility for any injury to people or property resulting from any ideas, methods, instructions or products referred to in the content.

www.ingramcontent.com/pod-product-compliance
Lightning Source LLC
LaVergne TN
LVHW072252110526
838202LV00106B/2597